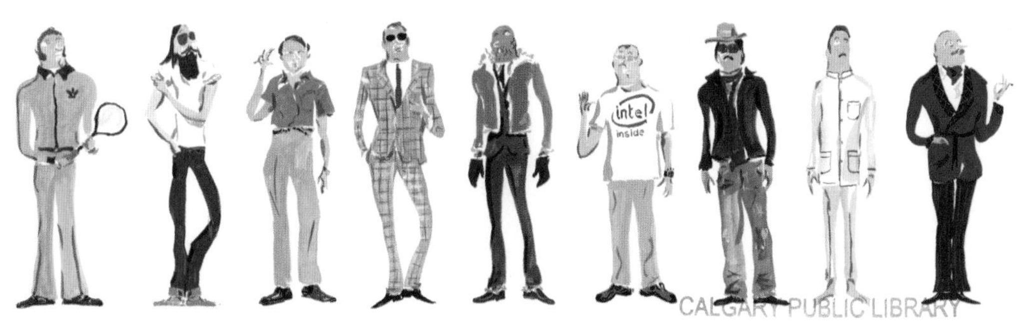
intel
inside

SUAVE

IN EVERY SITUATION

EDITORIAL DIRECTOR, FRENCH EDITION
Guillaume Robert

ENGLISH EDITION

EDITORIAL DIRECTOR
Kate Mascaro

EDITOR
Helen Adedotun

TRANSLATED FROM THE FRENCH BY
Jeanne B. Cheynel

COPYEDITING
Lindsay Porter

TYPESETTING
Claude-Olivier Four

PROOFREADING
Sam Wythe

COLOR SEPARATION
Bussière, Paris

PRINTED IN CHINA BY
Toppan Leefung

Originally published in French as
Comment rester chic en toutes circonstances

87, quai Panhard et Levassor
75647 Paris Cedex 13

editions.flammarion.com

17 18 19 3 2 1

ISBN: 978-2-08-020309-0

Legal Deposit: 03/2017

GONZAGUE DUPLEIX
JEAN-PHILIPPE DELHOMME

SUAVE

IN EVERY SITUATION

A Rakish Style Guide for Men

ART DIRECTOR
CELYA BENDJENAD

Flammarion
GQ

CONTENTS

When it comes to style, the world falls into two categories. There are people who just get it wrong, stubbornly maintaining that being suave is a bit like Tolkien's Mordor—a world of appearances as impenetrable and exhilarating as a VIP box. And then there are those like you and me, who believe, on the contrary, that elegance is a land full of mischief, a world of constant delight. Simple as that.

Gonzague Dupleix

I

ASK YOURSELF THE RIGHT

I —— 001 › I —— 028

What impact did World War I have on men's clothing? • What's a comb-over? • What do you use to wipe sand from your feet? • What sleepwear is right for you? • Whatever happened to the Kurt Cobain look? • Leather pants for all? • Is gingham ever cool? • When did cooks start wearing chef's hats? • Is it ok to put your feet up on the glove compartment? • Which shoe is the latest must-have? • Who started the slack necktie trend? • Should a man of style learn to sew? • Who is the real king of the jungle? • Is it ok to leave French cuffs unbuttoned? •

QUESTIONS

Are you a subway surfer? • Which boutonniere should you choose? • Can you wear a beret today? • Which French king introduced rigid rules of etiquette? • What is "camel toe"? • How can you spruce up small-town style? • When are hipsters unhip? • Are you ever too old to get a driver's license? • What is the latest fitness fad? • Does wearing a trench coat make you a gangster? • When did the first patterned socks appear? • Hip or hipster: can you spot the difference? • Should you wear your blazer inside out? • Can you flaunt a Gallic nose?

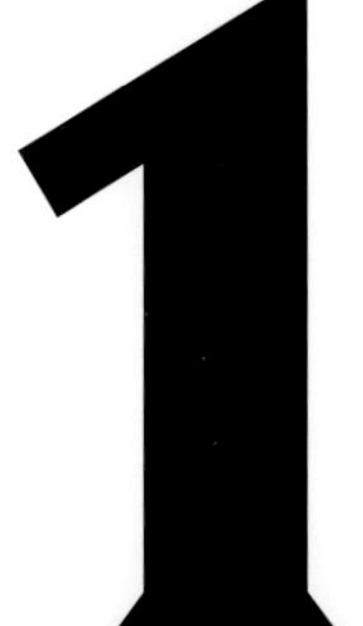

CHAPTER ONE

I —— 001

WHAT IMPACT DID WORLD WAR I HAVE ON MEN'S CLOTHING?

From 1914 to 1918, a fifth of the French population (eight million out of a total of forty million) was called to arms and into uniform. Following the armistice, a new world emerged. Dress codes changed. Accustomed to their uniforms, men switched to wearing functional, lighter-weight suits. The tuxedo, which debuted much earlier in the United States, now crossed the Atlantic to replace the frock coat. Diehard arbiters of style (who only experienced the war from their doorstep, of course) considered tuxedos inappropriate, likening them to a sort of society pajama. For all other explanations of the world's profound transformation, see French economist Thomas Piketty's book *Capital in the Twenty-First Century*—you'll devour two centuries of global economics as though you were savoring every word of a Balzac novel.

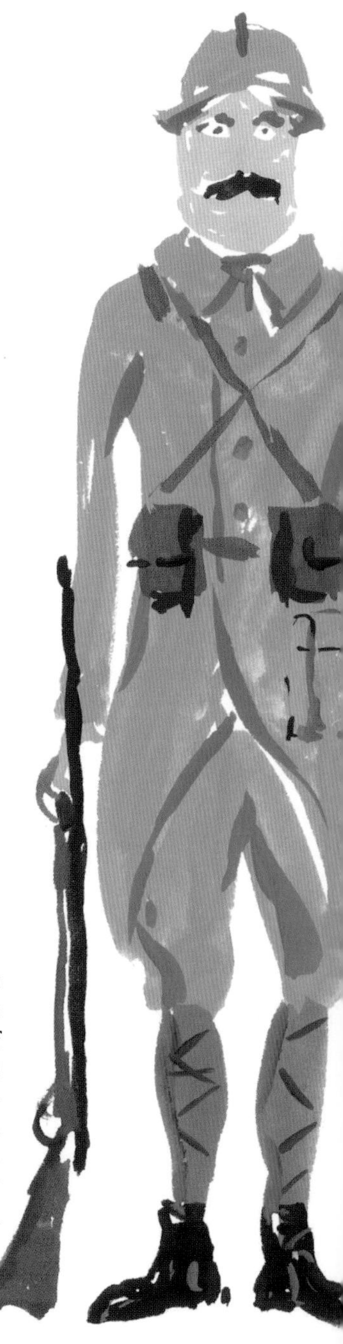

I —— 002

WHAT'S A COMB-OVER?

The comb-over, as seen on used-car salesmen everywhere, is a long flap of hair that sprouts from the temple. Those who refuse to embrace their baldness comb the hair over the top of their head. This hairstyle—the last bastion of an endangered virility, which can be swept away by the tiniest puff of wind—has become the centerpiece of identikit photos, along with those cheap, smoke-lens sunglasses you get at the drugstore. The comb-over is, distressingly, the elegant man's Achilles' heel. For decades, dubious remedies for baldness have been buried away, shamefully, in the back sections of men's magazines.

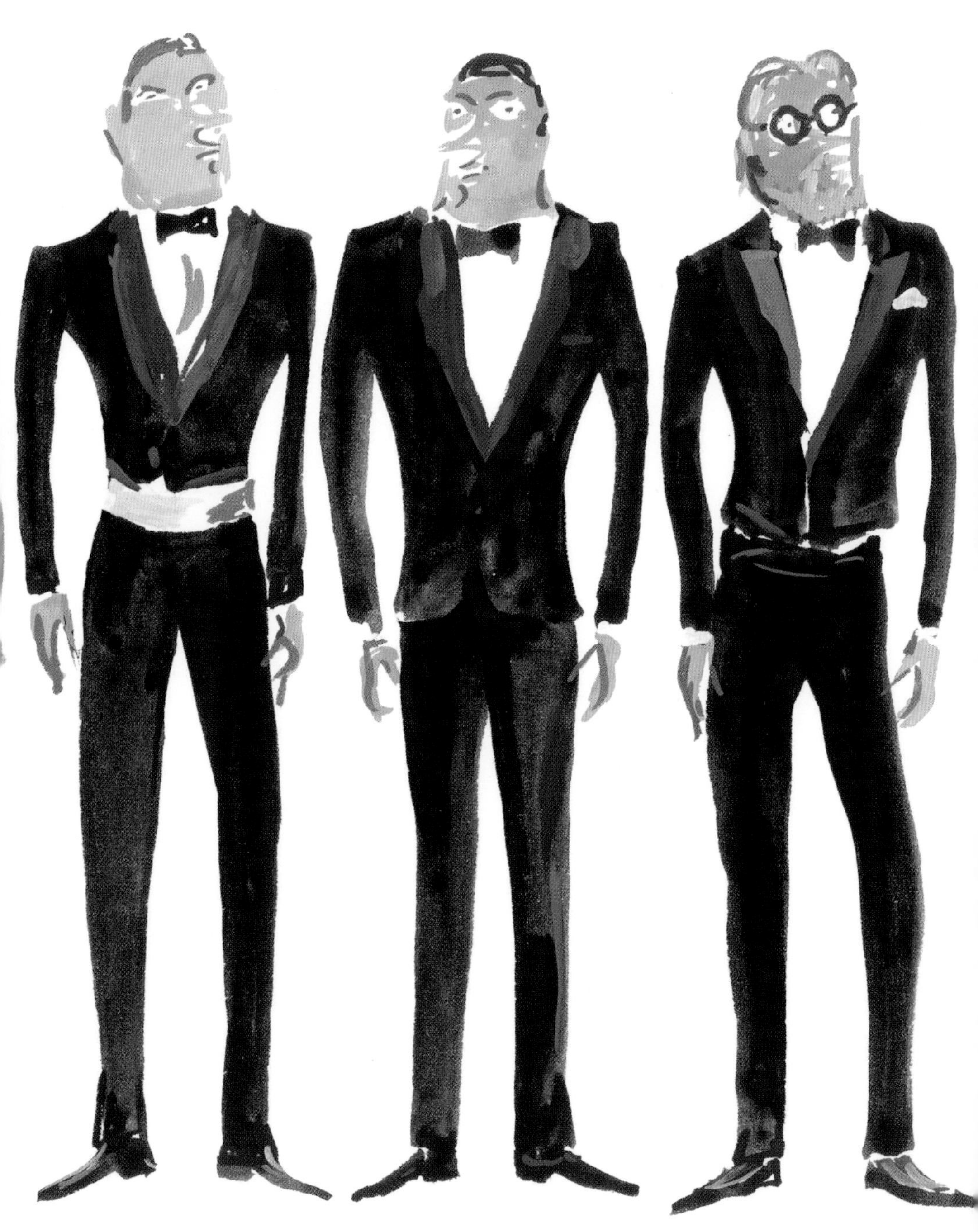

I —— 003

WHAT DO YOU USE TO WIPE SAND FROM YOUR FEET?

If you replied "hands," remind me not to shake yours. If you use your beach towel, shaken out beforehand, you might lack a certain creative flair, but at least the sand won't end its sorry existence in someone's eye. And of course, if you use a black biker bandanna, you'll look like a poser, but it will finally have served a useful purpose—something it has been desperately seeking for the last century.

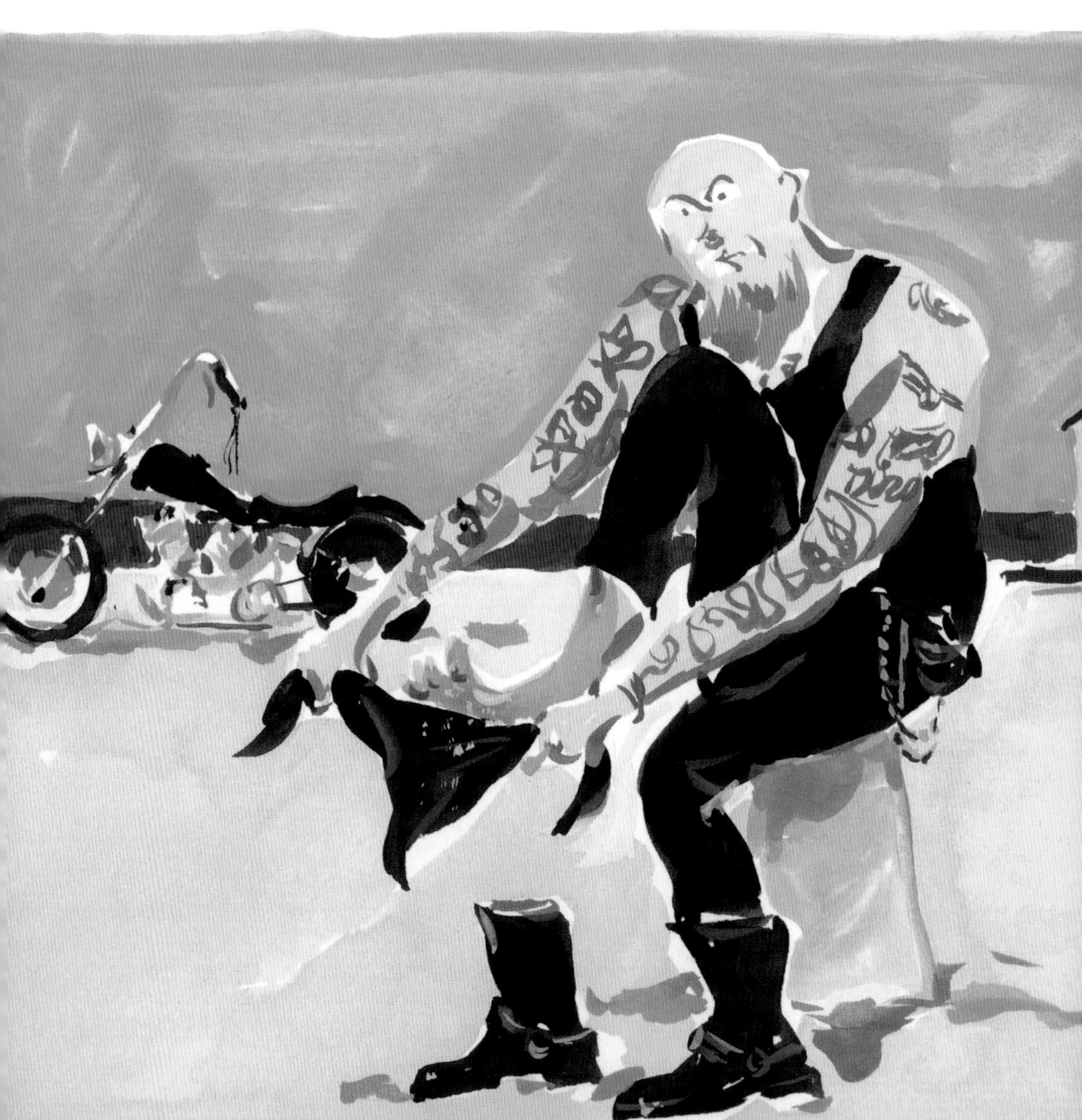

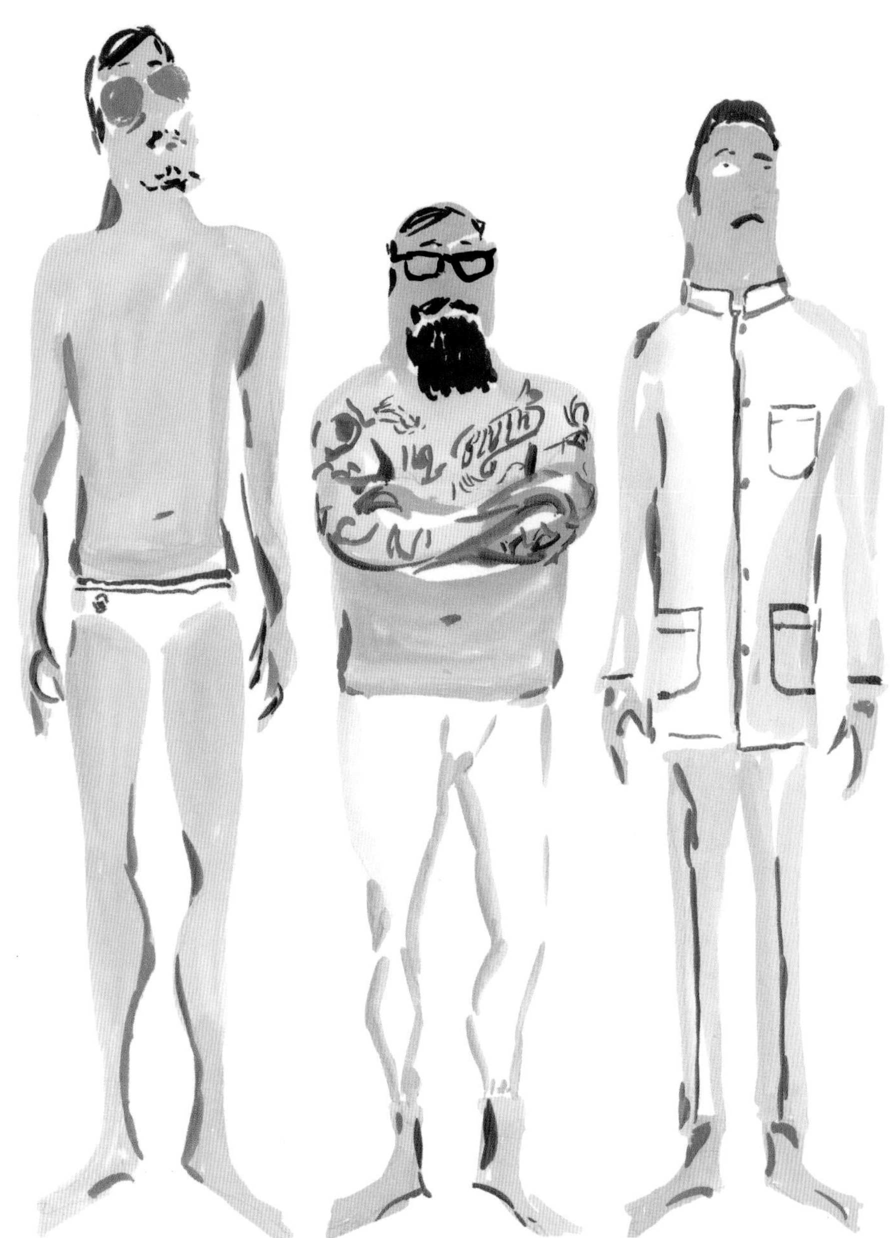

I —— 004

WHAT SLEEPWEAR IS RIGHT FOR YOU?

You've got three possibilities. 1. Your room is hot and so are you: sleep in classic *Risky Business* white briefs—nothing more, nothing less. 2. You're an adventurer, an outdoor type: thermals are good company. 3. You're a confirmed bachelor who doesn't like shapeless, straight pajamas: find a model with a mandarin collar. Though we adore briefs, we, too, prefer this last solution.

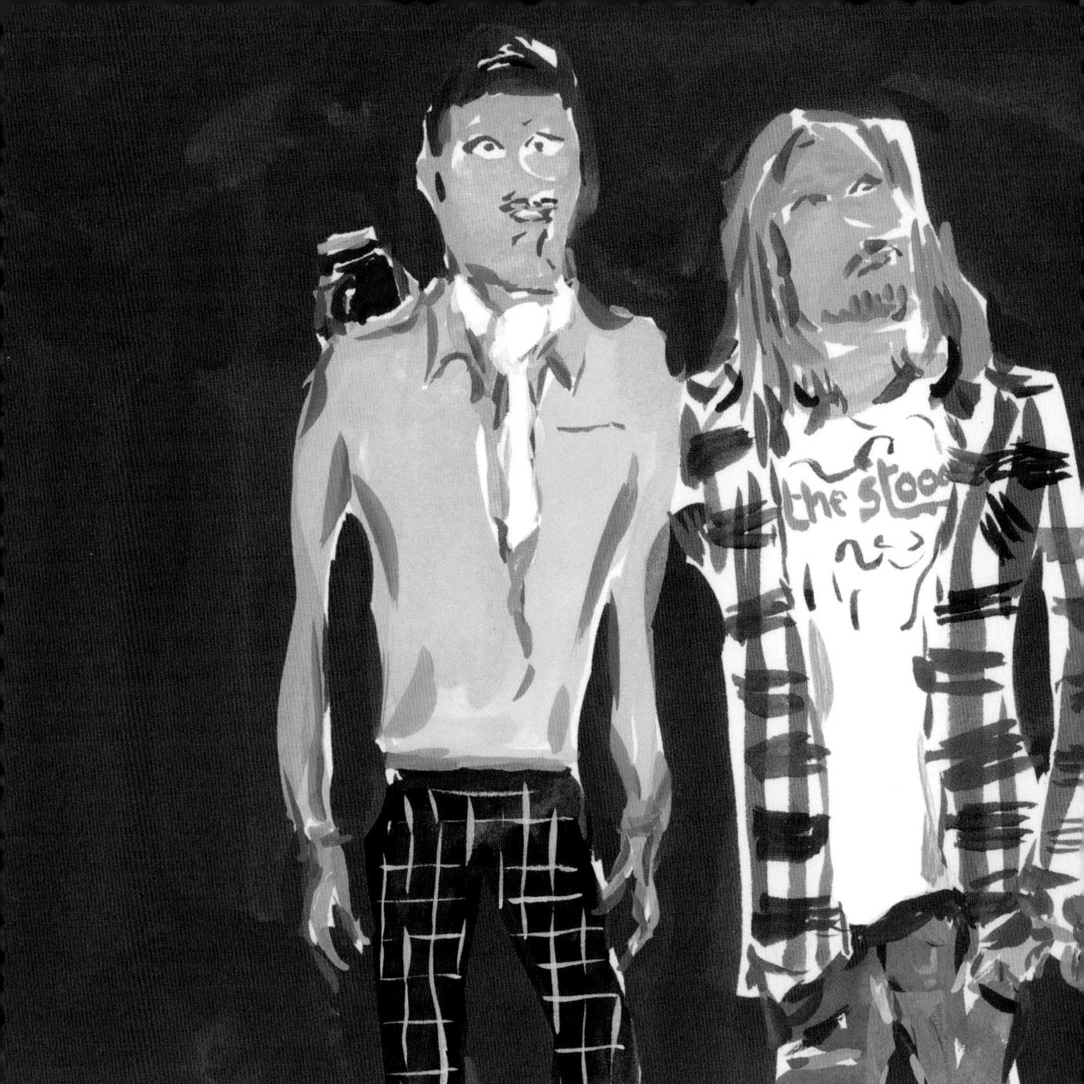

I —— 005

WHATEVER HAPPENED TO THE KURT COBAIN LOOK?

As we blow out the twenty or so candles on the monumental anniversary that marks his passing, what remains of Kurt Cobain's sartorial legacy? Just as Marlon Brando immortalized the black leather jacket (an item that simply ensured his safety when riding his motorcycle), Kurt Cobain sanctified the flannel shirt. He wore it over his favorite band T-shirt, like all the kids back then, basically to avoid freezing to death. Today, on the other hand, only the youngest can get away with ripped jeans. And just a handful of them, going for a low-tech nineties look (i.e., Windows 92), still color their hair at home. The ones who do a total bleach job—well, that's a whole different kettle of fish.

I —— 006

LEATHER PANTS FOR ALL?

Leather pants hugging the backsides of Patrick Swayze, John Lennon, Lou Reed, Alice Cooper, and Slash were smokin'. On Daft Punk's butts, pretty hot. More recently seen on Kanye West, they've gone room temp. In the early twenty-first century, leather pants have lost a bit of their S&M sizzle and are gradually going mainstream. Once they become available at affordable prices, it will be no surprise when kids under twenty-five make them popular again. After that, those with cash to splash—old thirty- and young fortysome-things—will wear them to look young and chic, with a white ruffled shirt just like Tom Jones in his prime.

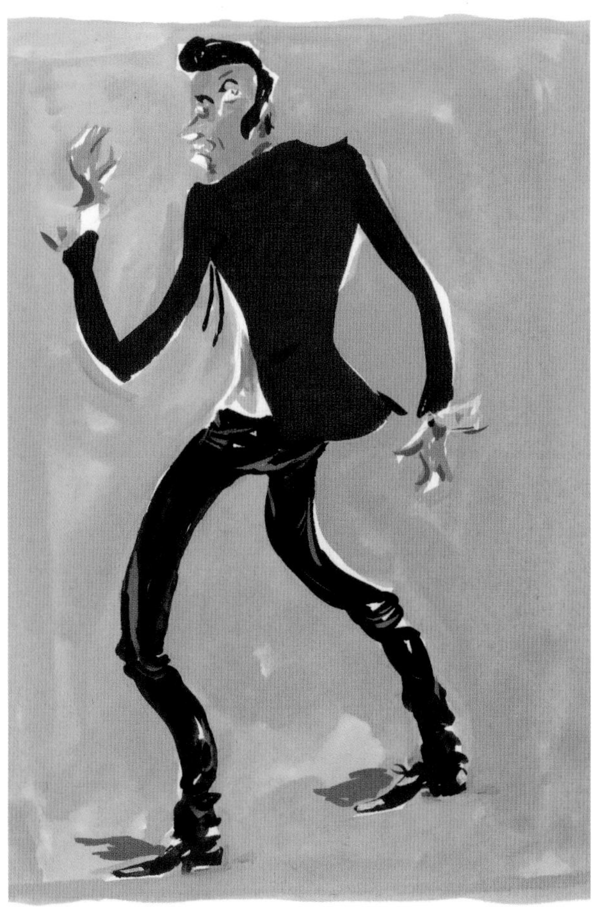

I —— 007

IS GINGHAM EVER COOL?

When Brigitte Bardot married Jacques Charrier in France in 1959, she wore a gingham dress. The wedding took place in Vichy, and the French name for this fabric was born. Gingham had been popular well before then, though; and while it was sweet and girlish in Victorian times, by the 1960s it was a sign of rebellion. Mods—stylish working-class teens in 1960s England—wore a dense blue-and-red version; bold and brash instead of dainty and demure. Americans now prefer a bigger print to go with a solid necktie for semi-formal situations. There you have it: the different connotations of gingham in three fine countries. Now you're free to adapt it to your own sartorial needs and desired effects.

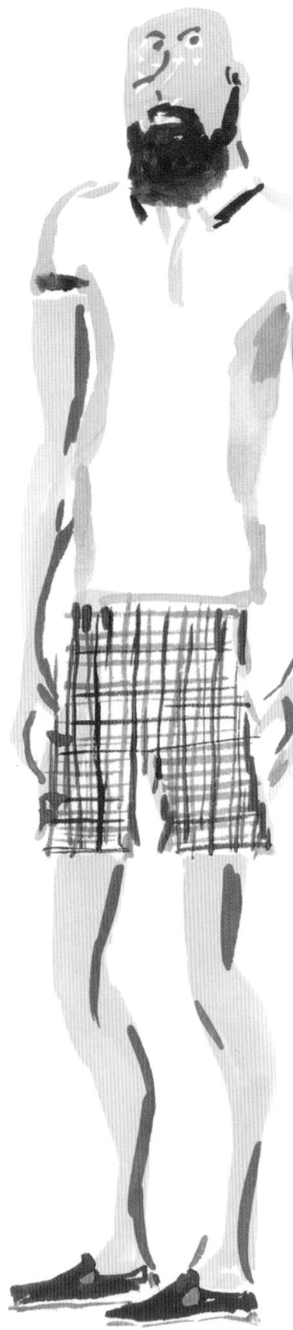

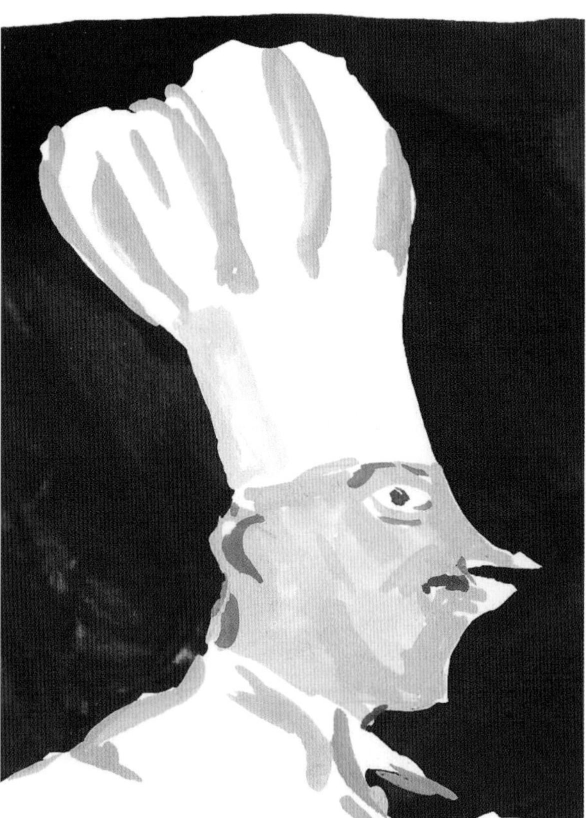

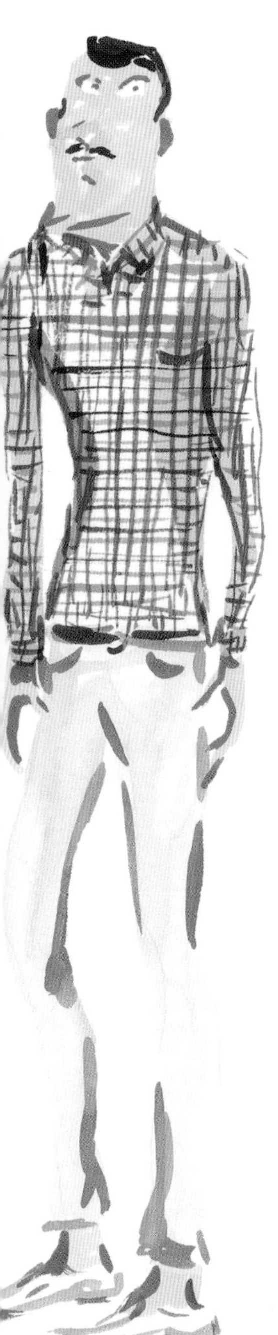

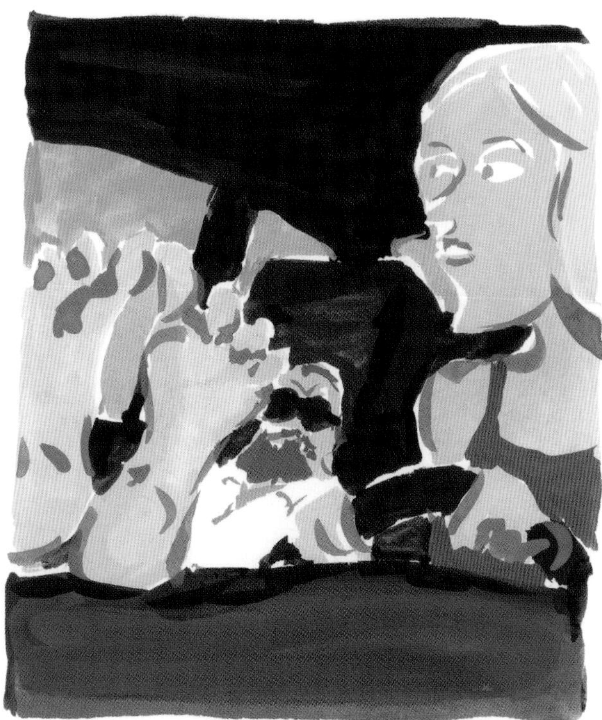

I —— 008

WHEN DID COOKS START WEARING CHEF'S HATS?

At the very beginning, cooks wore caps for hygienic reasons. Later, to distinguish the chefs from the kitchen boys, the caps came out in different heights. In the nineteenth century the chef's toque made its appearance (shout out to Marie-Antoine Carême, top of all the top chefs), which allowed the chef to keep a cool head in a hot kitchen. Once upon a time, the folds in the hat signified how many egg recipes the chef could cook.

I —— 009

IS IT OK TO PUT YOUR FEET UP ON THE GLOVE COMPARTMENT?

The road is long and your legs are numb. You, the passenger, liven up the trip by entertaining the driver with captivating conversation. If, after going to all this trouble, you don't have his consent to stretch your legs, just go ahead and assert your right to put your feet up—after having slipped on a fresh pair of socks, of course. In the event of a traffic jam, reposition yourself in your seat, your eyes fixed steadily ahead.

XX

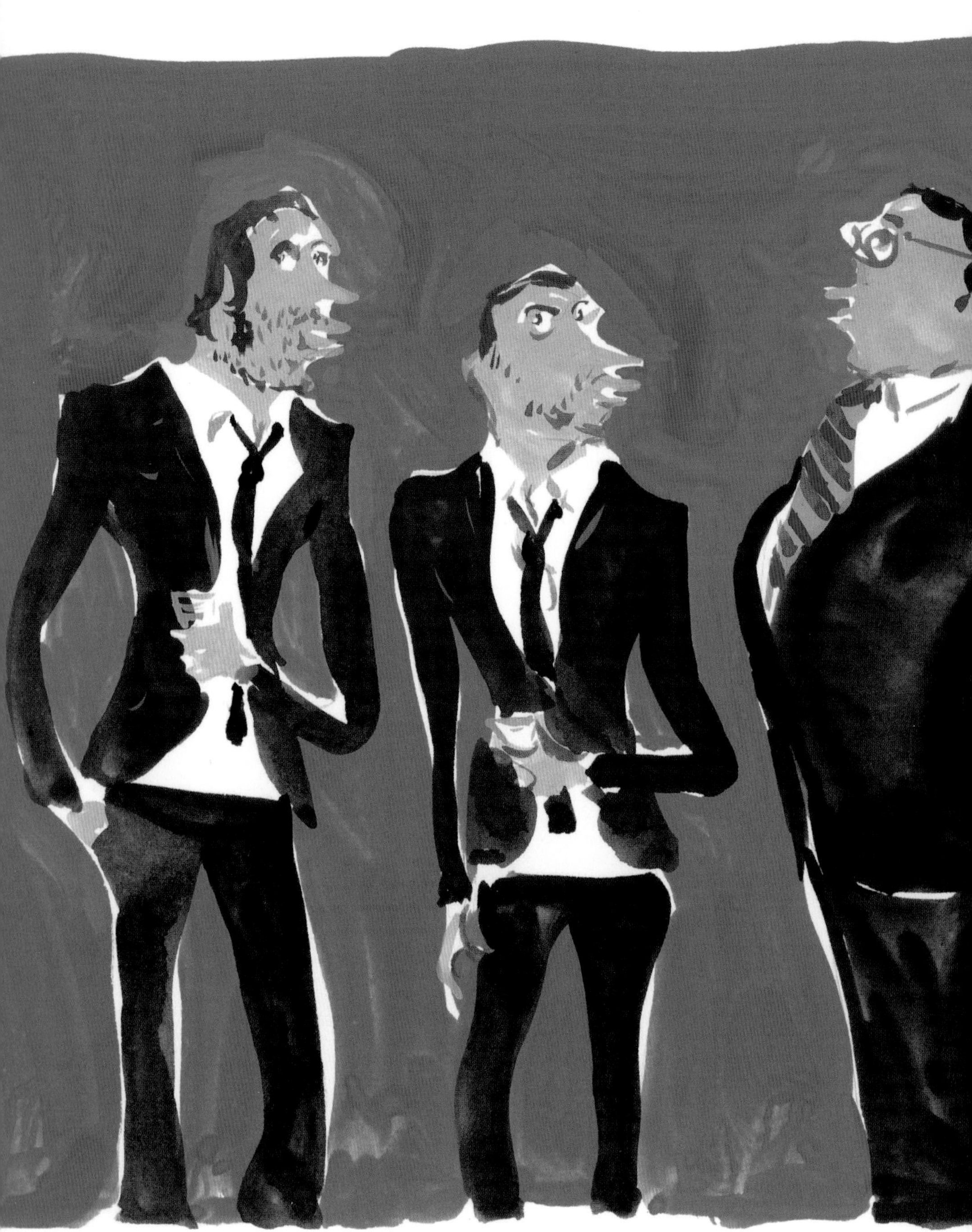

ASK YOURSELF THE RIGHT QUESTIONS

I — 010

WHICH SHOE IS THE LATEST MUST-HAVE?

Once upon a time, out on the playground, new white sneakers were made to be scuffed. Later, grownups who panicked at the first smudge were considered uptight losers, while world travelers sported the dirt as a badge of pride. New generation, new rules, and now the ultimate in cool is clean. Immaculate, box-fresh—today's casual shoe is whiter than white, a stranger to sports and the street—just like its wearer. For a living-on-the-edge look, he can outsource that spirit of adventure to someone else, and buy a "pre-worn" pair, brand new.

I — 011

WHO STARTED THE SLACK NECKTIE TREND?

The youngest among us (who think Peter Doherty invented it) and the oldest (who think Sinatra was its most zealous promoter) will be ticked off to learn that the first loose necktie appeared much earlier. According to a French fashion dictionary, in the late seventeenth century a dancer named Pécour left his collar ties undone while dancing a step called the chaconne. It became so fashionable, it inspired a loose necktie named after the dance.

I — 012

Should a man of style learn to sew?

Since life is pretty good and fashion diktats are relatively flexible, you don't have to pull out your sewing machine every two minutes. However, if you come across a vintage piece at the local secondhand store, or find something at the back of the closet that really could be something if given a little boost, or if you tear the lining of your jacket, a stitch in time truly will save nine. Knowing how to replace a missing shirt button can come in handy. Looking for a hobby? This is a good one.

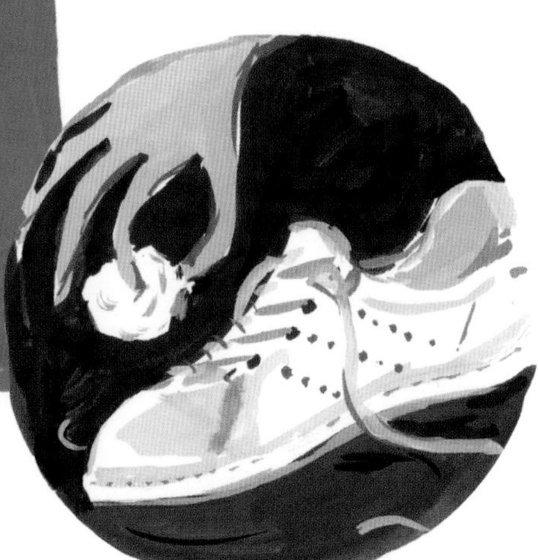

I —— 013

WHO IS THE REAL KING OF THE JUNGLE?

Ladies and gentlemen of the middle class, step right up: instead of the ubiquitous sheepskin collar, for a taste of the exotic the luxury industry now wants us to covet snakeskin. Your mission, should you choose to accept it, is to know how to wear it. Ankle boots and only ankle boots are the natural preference. But this is merely because the snakeskin jacket should be left to the professionals: Nicolas Cage in *Wild at Heart*, rapper Rick Ross, and the Lizard King himself, Jim Morrison. At least we can get a kick out of seeing a slithering creature transformed into a hustler shoe. More and more, men's fashion is leading us into disco funk land, where, without a second thought, honest men aspire to look like small-time crooks, drug dealers, and pimps. There are many reasons for this, not least the fact that as gentrification is replacing actual urban grit we're happy to play at being edgy, without actually living on the edge.

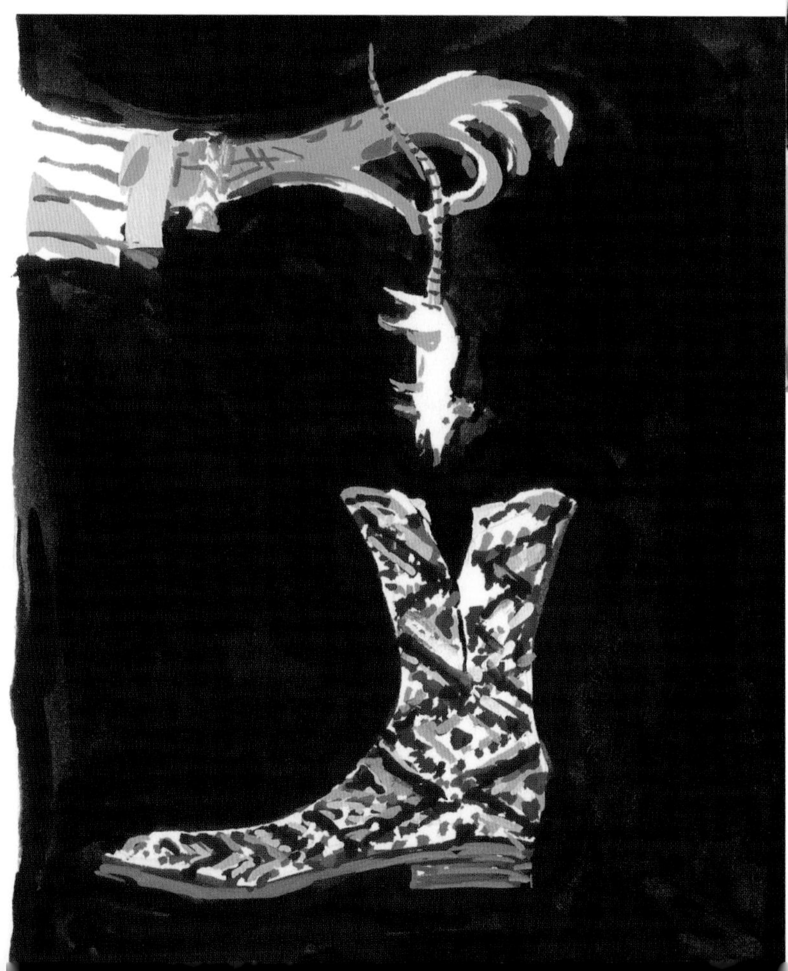

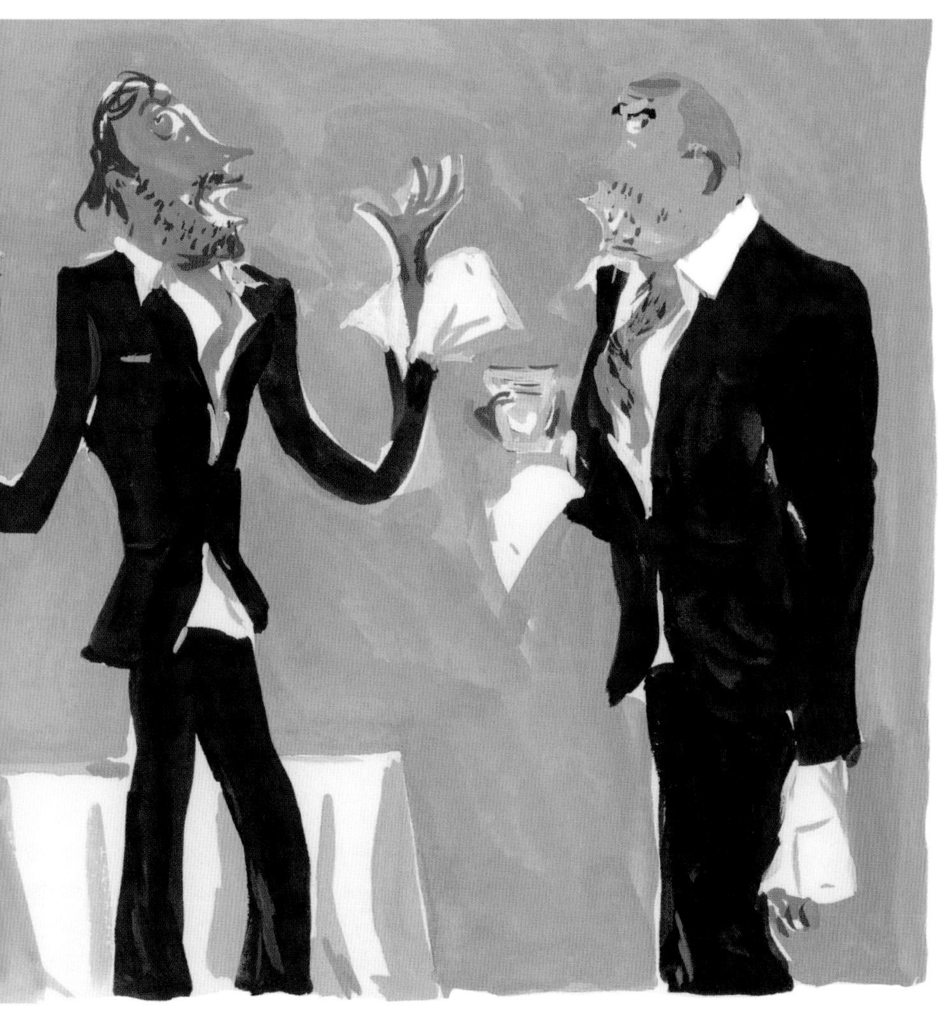

I —— 014

IS IT OK TO LEAVE FRENCH CUFFS UNBUTTONED?

This sexy, disheveled, Left Bank French look was in style in the late 1990s, and it still is among a certain kind of eternal-dandy, loud-mouthed, velvet-jacketed thirtysomething with philosophical pretensions. It has the disadvantage of swallowing up the hand. It's better to leave your cuffs unbuttoned only when you're seated and need to use your hands to talk: if you're standing up, your arms will look short and you won't look quite so clever. Trying to eat *œufs mayonnaise* with them unbuttoned is an entirely different matter.

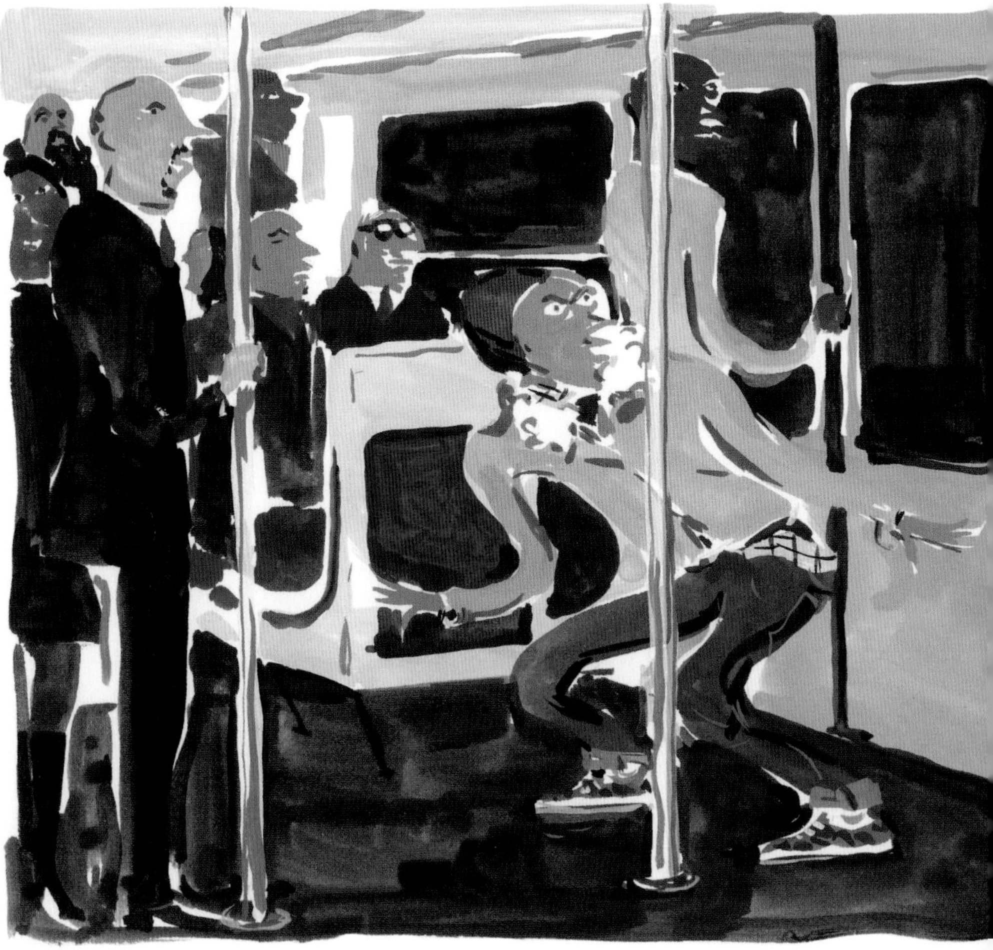

1 —— 015

ARE YOU A SUBWAY SURFER?

Guys who always act surprised when the subway jolts as the train speeds forward are like people who never remember what they've ordered in a restaurant. You, on the other hand, with your feet parallel to one another and in line with the longitudinal axis of the rails, your thighs ever so slightly bent, never have to hang onto the central support bar. Shift your weight to your front foot before the subway comes to a halt; shift your weight toward the back when the train starts to pull forward again: you won't look clueless, you'll look—and rightly so—like a winner. When seated, don't even think about manspreading; no gentleman would ever do that in public.

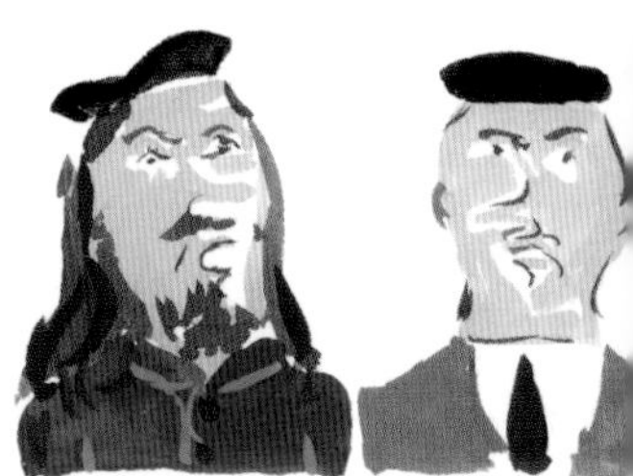

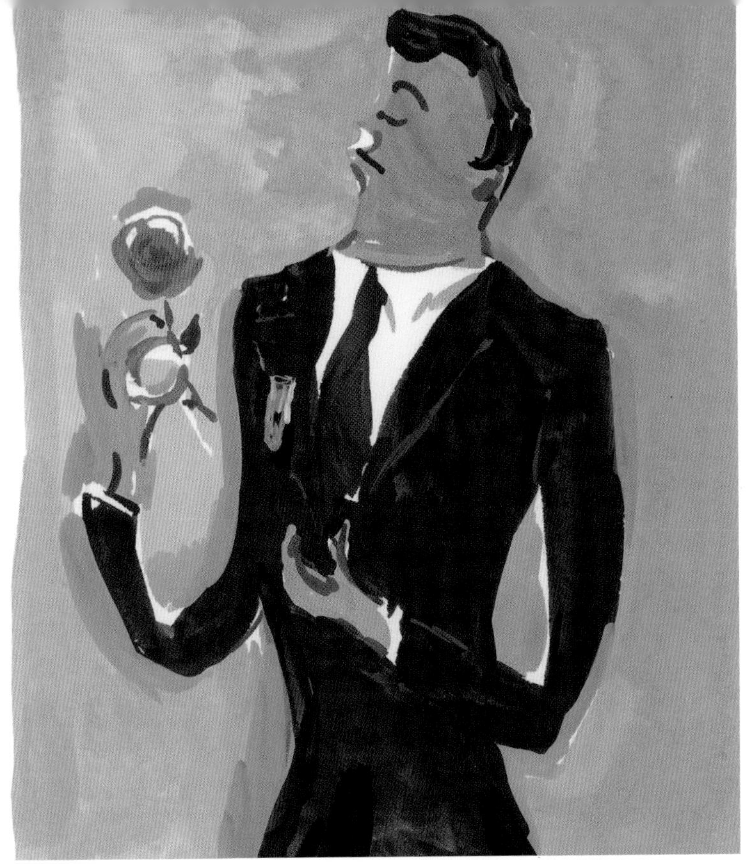

I —— 016

WHICH BOUTONNIERE SHOULD YOU CHOOSE?

Hallmark of formalwear, the boutonniere—sometimes inserted into a mini vase to keep it fresh on your lapel—is typically a simple rose. But let's take a minute for a brief history lesson on the language of flowers. In contrast to revolutionary red, the white fleur-de-lis was the official symbol of royalty in France from the time of Henry IV. In World War I, young recruits wore sky-blue uniforms and the French wear a commemorative cornflower today, much like the Remembrance Day poppy worn in the Commonwealth. Marcel Proust was more taken with camellias, and Oscar Wilde's favorite was a green carnation. Consider yourself instructed.

I  017

CAN YOU WEAR A BERET TODAY?

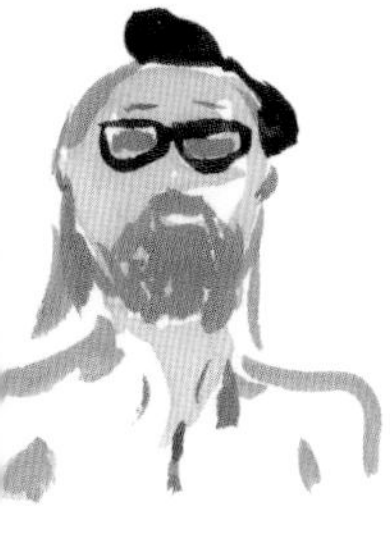

Rub your eyes as long as you'd like, because you're not seeing things: traditional berets are back. Mention of this typically French hat calls to mind, in no particular order, Field Marshal Montgomery, Samuel L. Jackson, Saddam Hussein, the Black Panthers, Jimmy Cliff, and Che Guevara. To get your bearings among this pantheon of panache, consider this: wear the beret to the right, you're in the company of defenders and heroes; to the left, you're among poets; in the middle—you just look dumb.

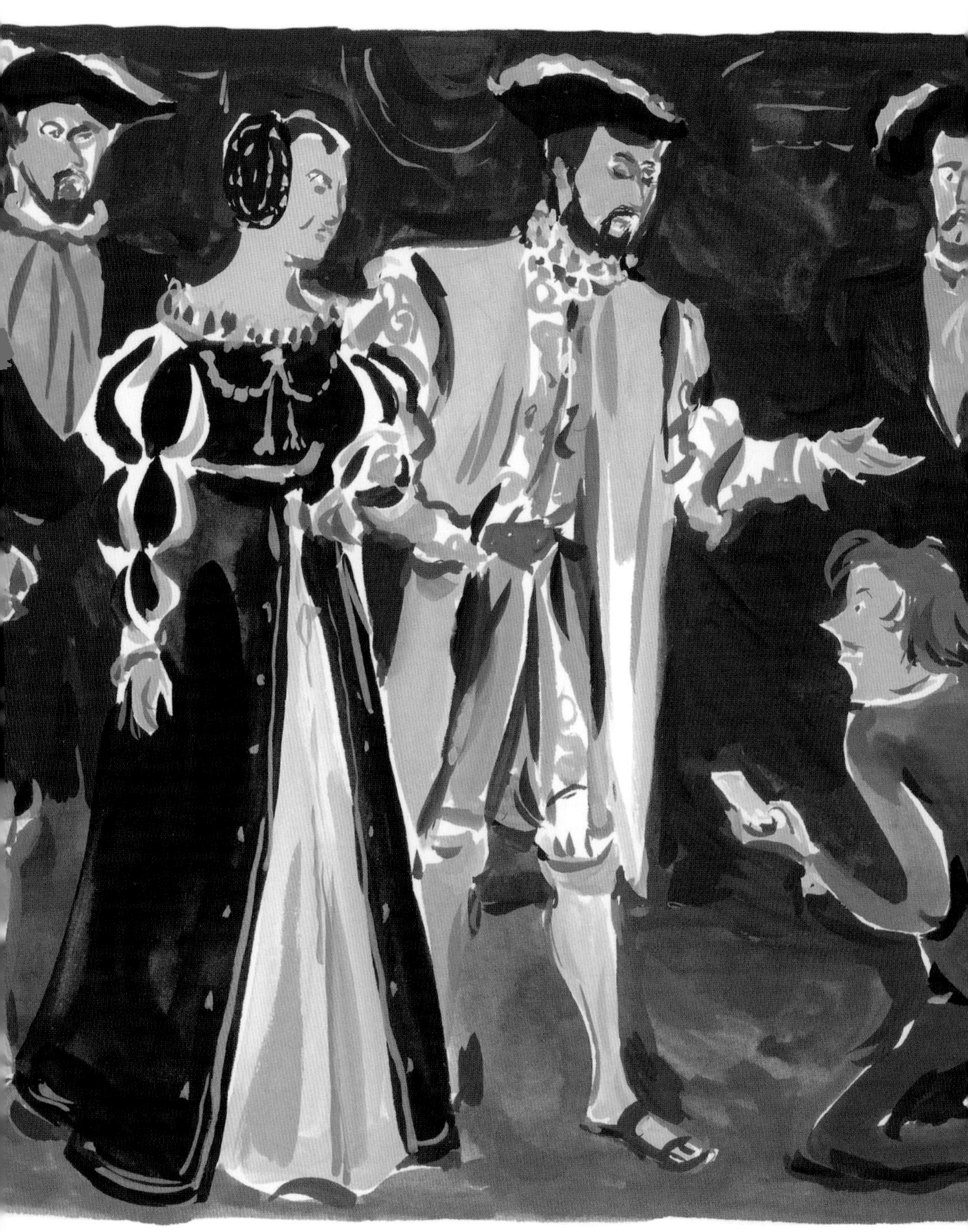

ASK YOURSELF THE RIGHT QUESTIONS

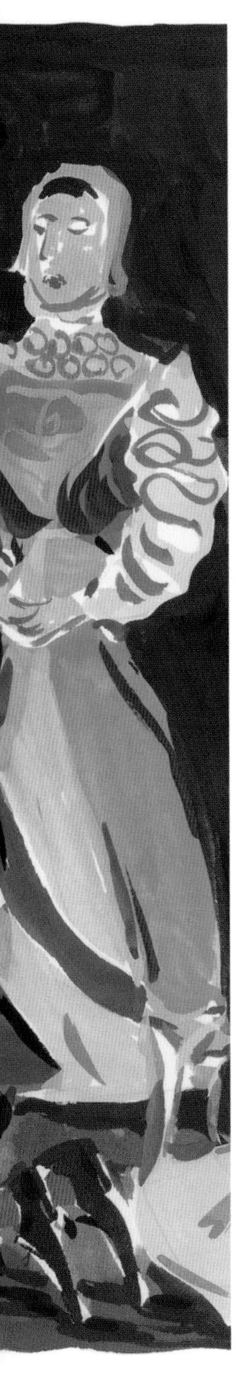

I —— 018

WHICH FRENCH KING INTRODUCED RIGID RULES OF ETIQUETTE?

One Sunday morning in March, we galloped through the Château de Blois in France's Loire Valley. We were alone and sped from room to room as though the future of France depended on it. We even climbed down the stairway to the Estates General room, feeling as though an imaginary court were observing us (in actual fact, a family was there, taking selfies on a cardboard throne). In the sixteenth century, such behavior would have displeased Renaissance king Henry III, who first codified life at court, shattering the bonhomie of human relations among the powerful.

I —— 019

What is "camel toe"?

Not just a female fashion faux pas, "camel toe"—when too-tight pants pinch your privates—can also strike men if they wear loose boxer shorts under tight-fitting jeans and the seam divides the area concerned into two equal parts. Fortunately for us, a simple solution to this unpleasant contemporary phenomenon exists—a good old pair of briefs, and that's that.

I —— 020

HOW CAN YOU SPRUCE UP SMALL-TOWN STYLE?

By going with the flow. You would be surprised to note that a young, dynamic executive from, say, North Platte, Nebraska, has the same look as a security guard in New York State. To show others you've seen a bit of the world, don't rush to buy the latest trends in the major chain stores. And don't clean out the small shops that sell last season's looks. Don't get caught in a trap. Hone your judgment, then adapt your wardrobe to the man you think you are. Find your own twist (or signature). Finally, make use of the right fashion tics at the right time: slim fit—out; plaid shirts—still around, but you should tread lightly; men's capri pants—out of the question. And so on. Understand that street style feeds fashion, particularly if it's down and dirty. And don't worry: sooner or later your style will be in.

I —— 021

WHEN ARE HIPSTERS UNHIP?

For crying out loud. For the past five years, you've had an Amish beard, tattoos to rival a Russian convict, and you dress like a Canadian trapper. How did this happen, you ask yourself. Burned out, you recently began longboarding to find a new meaning to your life. The result was a total flop. Endlessly listening to Tame Impala didn't exactly help matters, either. For a start at salvation, try shaving. Next, open your closet to the exotic patterns and warm colors that you lack. Get rid of the cap, plaid shirt, and work boots, and stop rolling up the cuffs of your jeans. Finally, find a pair of trousers that fits and everything will be hunky-dory again.

I —— 022

ARE YOU EVER TOO OLD TO GET A DRIVER'S LICENSE?

The law makes no mention of this subject. So the question is, just how long are you going to continue to pester your friends into giving you a ride, as though you were still twelve-and-a-half and had to get to ping-pong practice?

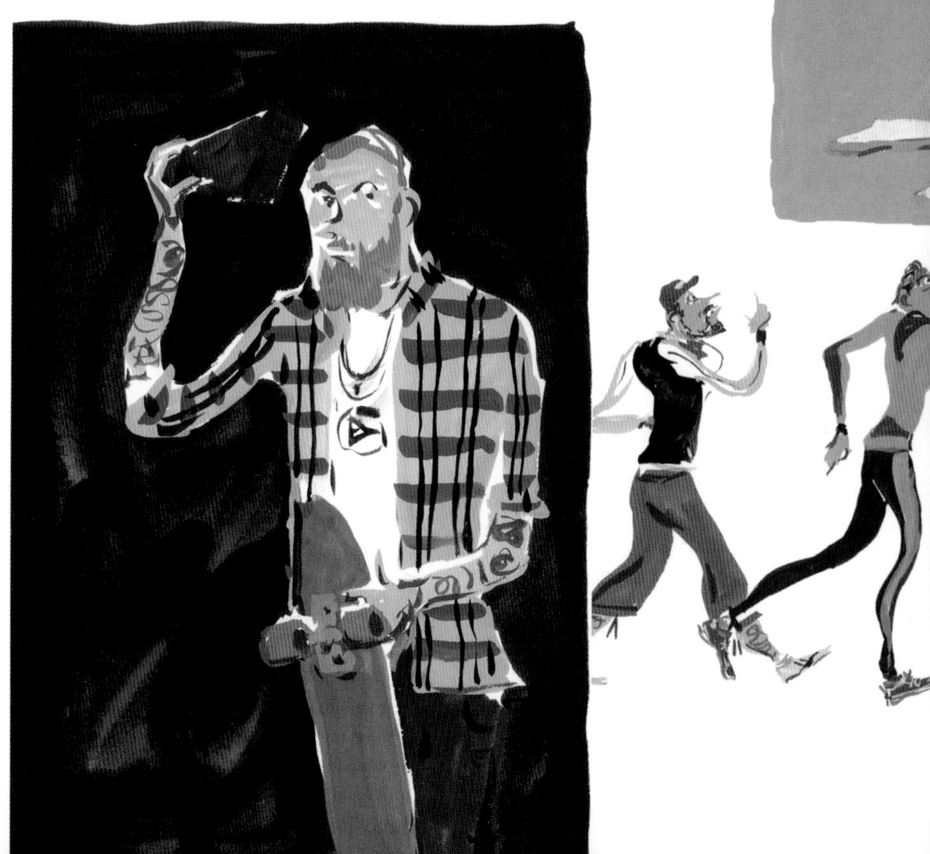

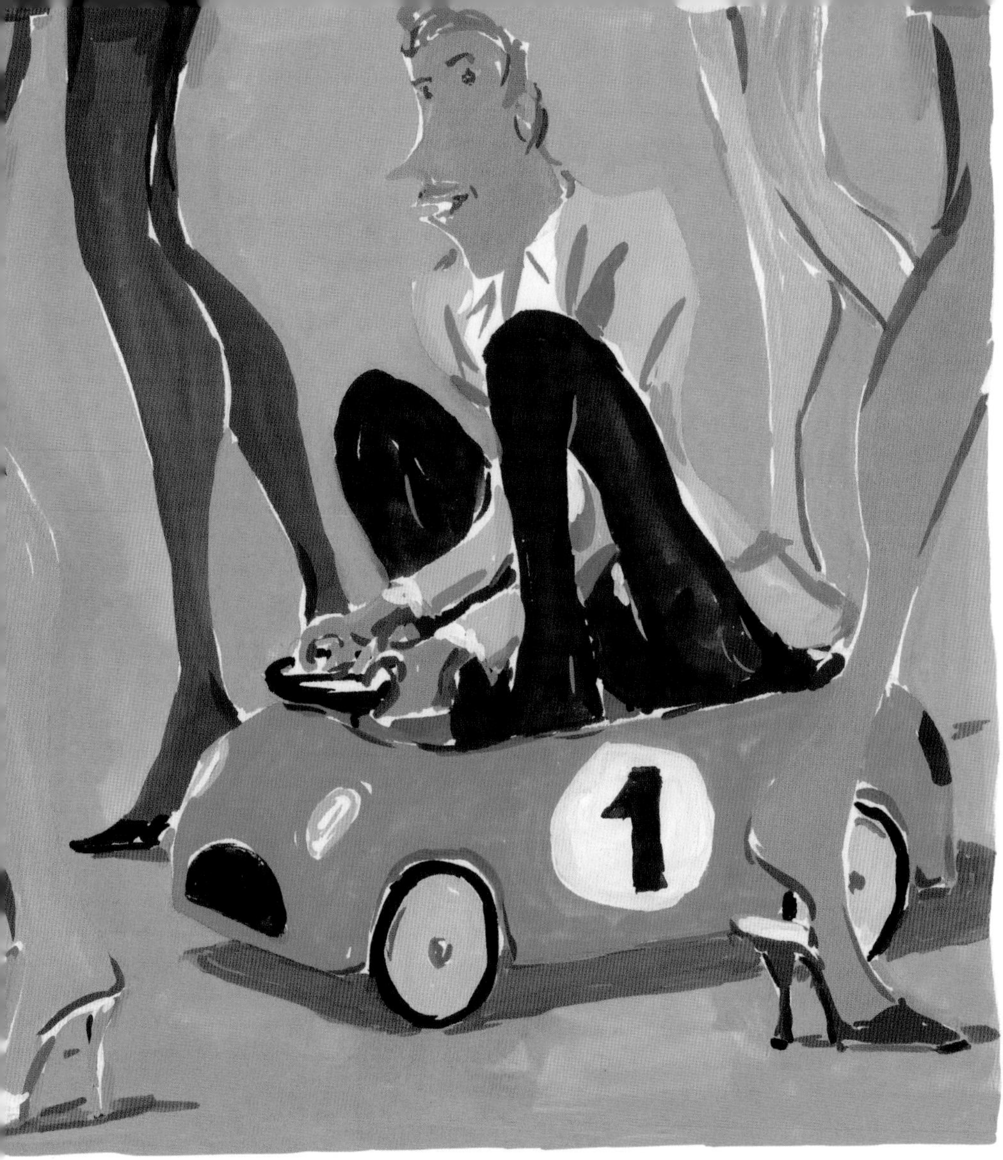

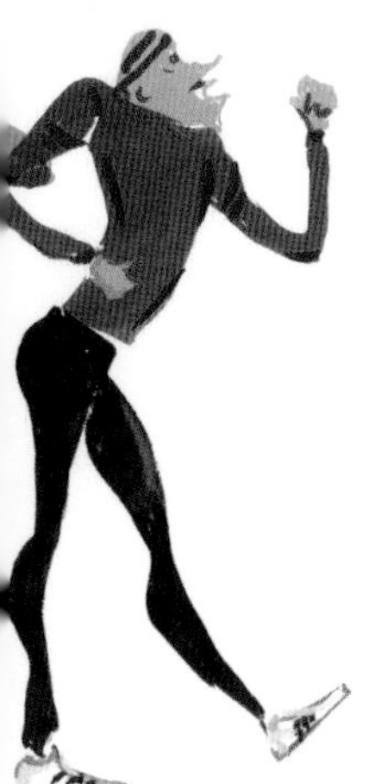

I —— 023

WHAT IS THE LATEST FITNESS FAD?

Do you feel torn between cycling, which is currently booming, and jogging, which is a little, shall we say, predictable? If so, start race walking. Very strange looking because of its stiff, swinging movements, this physical activity nevertheless demands total self-control. When it comes to the outfit, though, it requires a total lack of pride, which is why it fascinates us. Do not hesitate to go for any synthetic fabric possible and to choose short, loose cuts for ease of movement, as well as stirrup pants. You'll have us in tears of admiration—almost.

I —— 024

DOES WEARING A TRENCH COAT MAKE YOU A GANGSTER?

Designed during World War I as a solution to bad weather on battlefields, trench coats identify men who like to think they dice with death. Roomy and long, in Al Capone's Chicago they were ideal for hiding a sawn-off shotgun and other tools of the gangster's trade, especially on days when the sun was scarce. Over time, trench coats became the favorite clothing item of poets, punks, goths, new wavers—and flashers, of course. Despite all this, many men consider it the perfect overcoat for arriving on time—if not first—for a Monday morning meeting. What a crime.

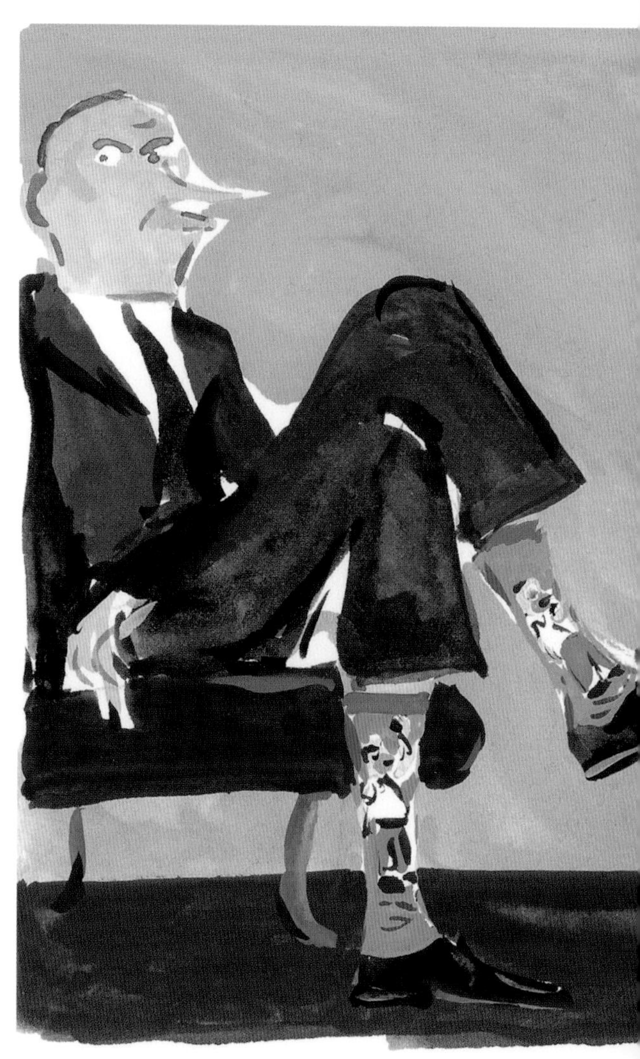

I —— 025

When did the first patterned socks appear?

Socks became standardized, comfortable, and elasticized in the 1940s. Prior to that, they were knitted and had to be held up with garters, which often failed, leaving men to yank them up, unwittingly revealing their socks. It was only logical that fancy patterns and artificial colors should follow. Until they have a complete makeover, today fancy socks are totally taboo.

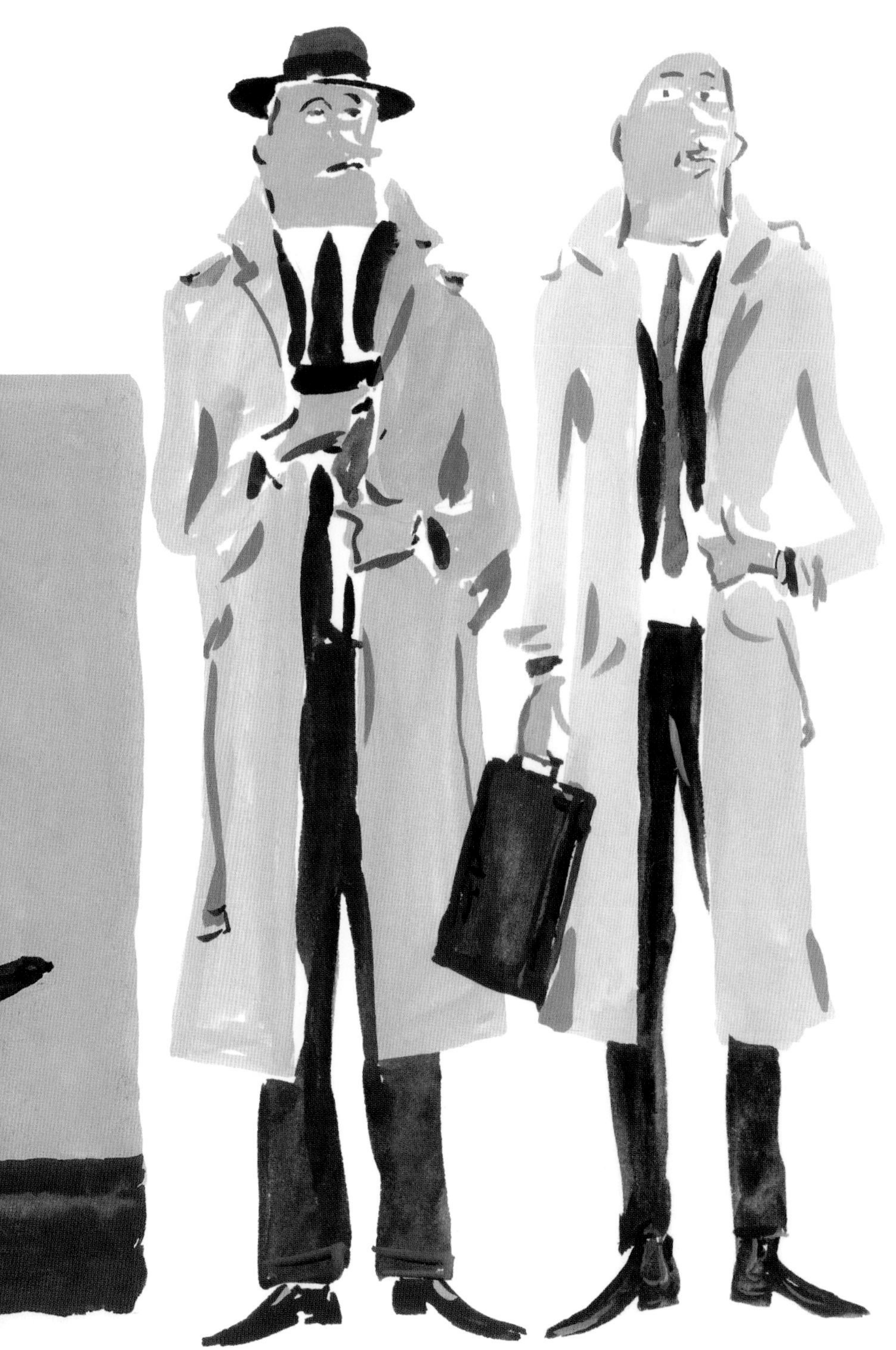

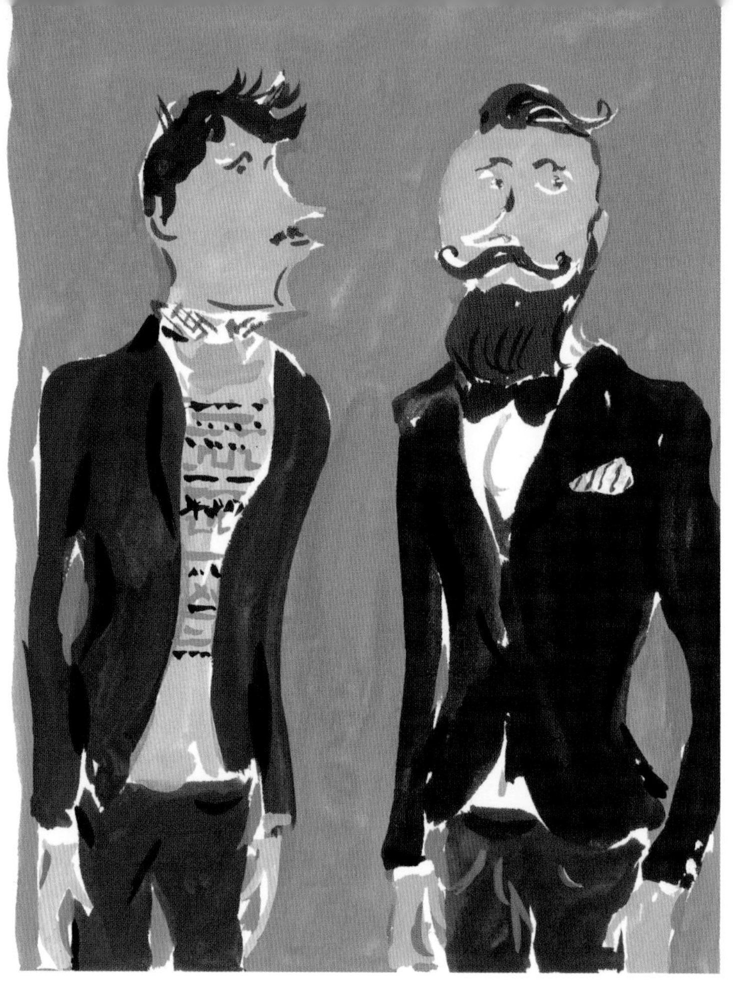

1 —— 026

HIP OR HIPSTER: CAN YOU SPOT THE DIFFERENCE?

To the naked eye, a hip person out and about has visibly wilder body hair than the hipster, who looks disciplined and openly well-groomed in terms of what he snips, smoothes, and coifs. Just shy of being totally bohemian, the perennially hip man makes a point of rubbing out any trace that could link him to a bathroom. His thing is to sleep while standing; his Holy Grail, to breeze in like the guy whose night was so wild that it makes everyone jealous. That's why he always seems to be coming down from a night of wild lovemaking and on the verge of a barbershop appointment that never happens. A hipster, on the other hand, does his utmost to look sharp. His clothes are as impeccable as they were in the shop window, and his hair as silky as in his Tinder profile pic. If you see a hipster wearing a rolled wool beanie, it's because his efforts have at last paid off and he's finally been successful at staying out all night.

I —— 027

SHOULD YOU WEAR YOUR BLAZER INSIDE OUT?

Will Smith was so cool that he'll doubtless be given credit for originating this style in *The Fresh Prince of Bel-Air* (we sort of suspect our American college friends knew the trick beforehand, but we can't find any evidence). There's no point in mimicking it in your daily life. But let's not be too sectarian: even though it might expose you to serious sanctions, giving a new twist to a uniform is still possible. To do so, you need to be in a very strict boarding school, where you're bored to death, and where you need to find way to let yourself go from time to time, to the delight of your ultra-privileged peers. Then don't forget to highlight your look with a lock of hair that dangles negligently into the right eye.

I —— 028

Can you flaunt a Gallic nose?

Since the nose serves as HQ for the sense of smell, ruling intuition and the emotions, it plays a very important role in helping to define a man's character. A prominent nose signifies a big personality, and gives you a regal profile like the kings of France. Voilà. The history of France—which sometimes offers an alibi for people who are in trouble—has come to your rescue. Lord it over the button-nosed.

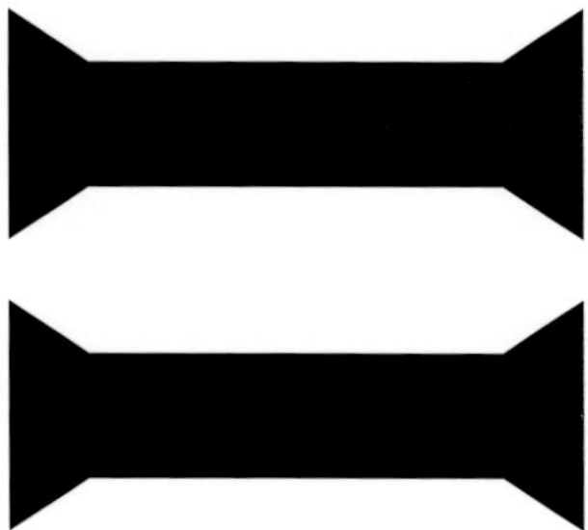

FOOL WITH

II —— 001 › II —— 013

Should you throw rice at a wedding? • How do you eat, drink, and be suave? • What look can you steal from Michel Houellebecq? • How can you avoid looking vacuum-packed? • Should you pick a strand of hair off someone's shoulder? • How do you freshen up clothes that reek of cheese fondue? • Boxers or briefs? • Can a gentleman wear sports paraphernalia with

THE RULES

a suit? • Why is chivalry dead? • Have scallops gone fishy? • At the movies, when is the right moment to plunge your hand into the popcorn? • What are the ten steps to normcore? • Can you let it all hang out when hanging out in the locker room?

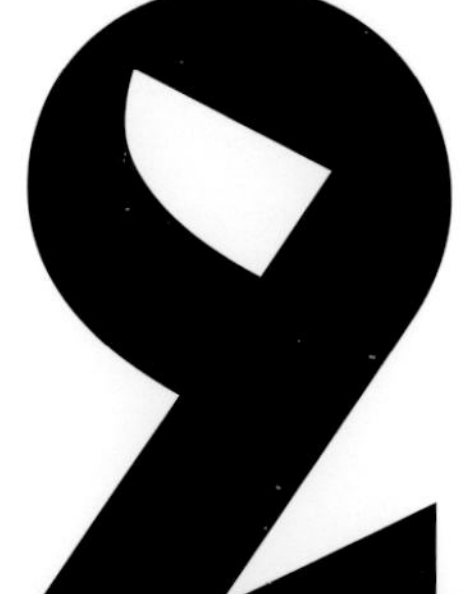

CHAPTER TWO

II —— 001

SHOULD YOU THROW RICE AT A WEDDING?

You can be sure that we have good reason to advise against this, despite the full weight of superstition and class ritual behind it. However, since we don't want to keep harking back to the past when making judgment calls, we've given the question some thought, using our characteristic common sense. To us, it seems that tossing rice into the bride's and groom's hair is tantamount to a cowardly variation of photobombing—a highly amusing practice that consists in ruining another person's photo in the most imaginative way possible. For this reason we don't condone rice throwing—it just lacks flamboyance. In addition, rice isn't all that photogenic: not only does it cause the person who gets hit in the face to wince, but it also ruins the outfit of a lifetime.

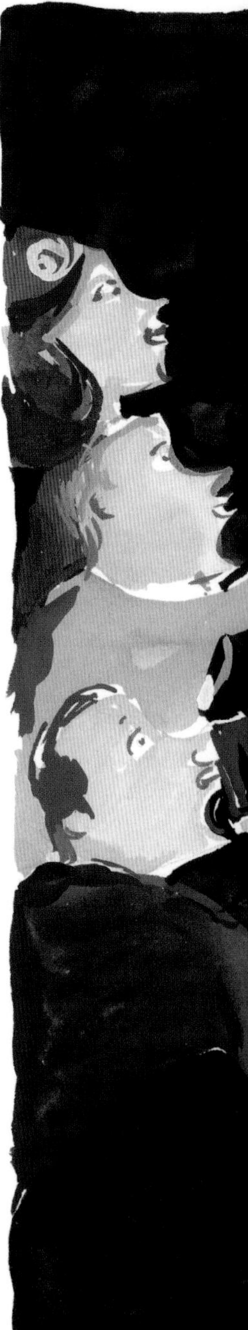

II —— 002

HOW DO YOU EAT, DRINK, AND BE SUAVE?

1. This isn't about grabbing a bite, unwrapping a sandwich at your desk, or, god forbid, eating while you walk. To dine is a verb. Give it some respect. 2. At the table, you are the director of drinks, so make sure everyone has one. It's surprising how many people never think of it. 3. Before you are even asked, pass around the bread basket, the salt, the pepper, or the salad bowl, reserving a look for anyone who grabs it from you without a thank-you. 4. Discreetly ask someone to pass you what you want and thank them, without interrupting the flow of conversation. Do *not* lean across the table to grab a piece of bread, even though other members of your party may be doing so. 5. And of course, leave your cell phone in your pocket—on silent—and do not envy those who place theirs next to their plate.

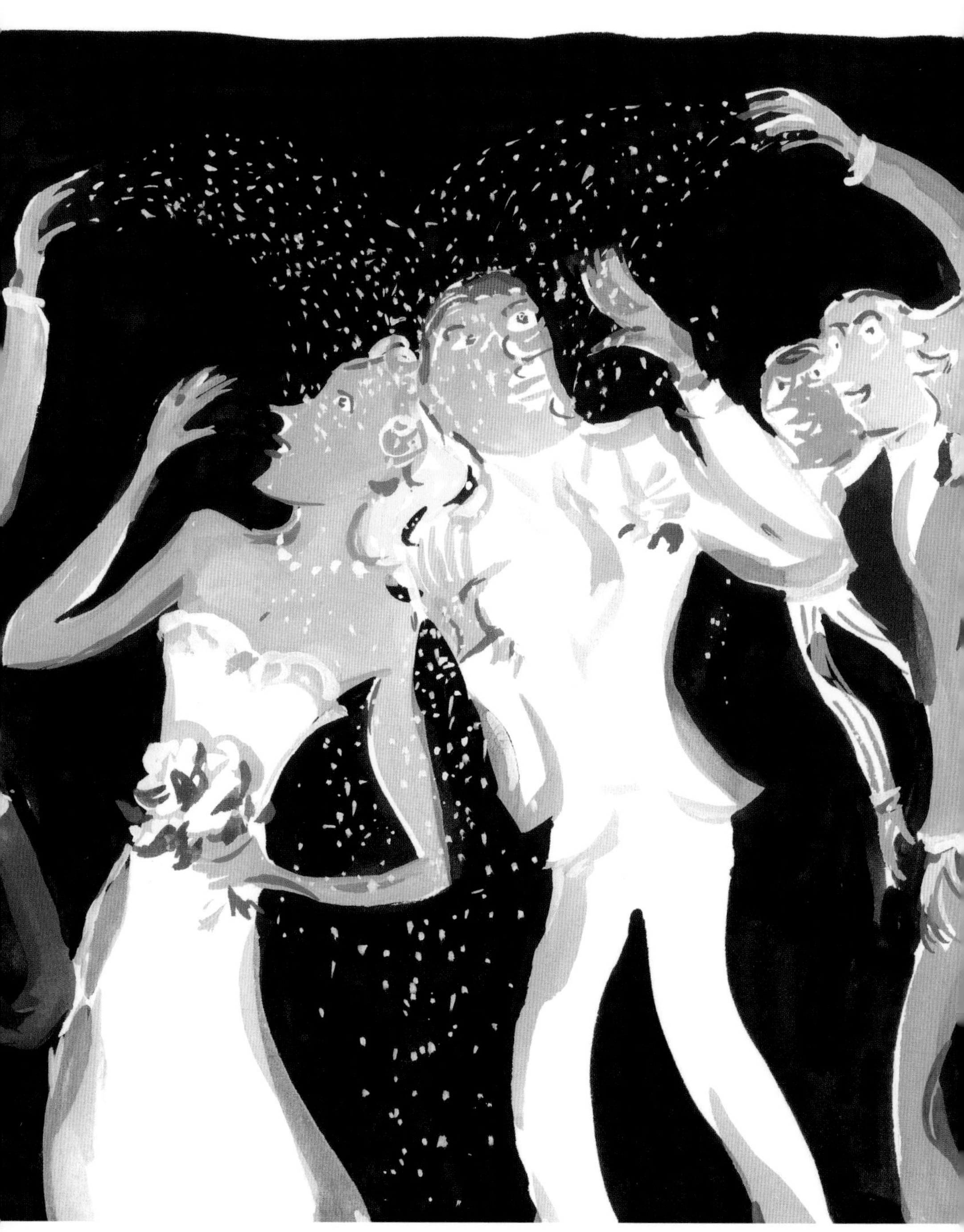

II —— 003

WHAT LOOK CAN YOU STEAL FROM MICHEL HOUELLEBECQ?

We'll leave literary style out of it here, to focus on the man. From your washing machine, take out an indigo shirt of denim, chambray, or cotton, with a button-down collar, and put it on a hanger to dry. Then wear it as is, or press it with an unplugged iron. Avoid touching the collar at all costs—it must curl up at the edges. Wear the shirt with pleated chinos—more daring than brown corduroys—a parka with a collar that you can roll the hood into, a round gold watch with a braided band, and a pair of Paraboot, Hush Puppies, or any other outdated brand of orthopedic shoe, such as the unparalleled Dr. Scholl slip-on. It's simple—just wear the best of the worst fashion picks. This is precisely why, little by little, these pieces come back into style.

II —— 004

How can you avoid looking vacuum-packed?

Being the fine observer that you are, you will have noted that the body has a tendency to look like a stuffed sausage when clothes are too small. Choose a size that allows room for "an invisible hand" to slip inside.

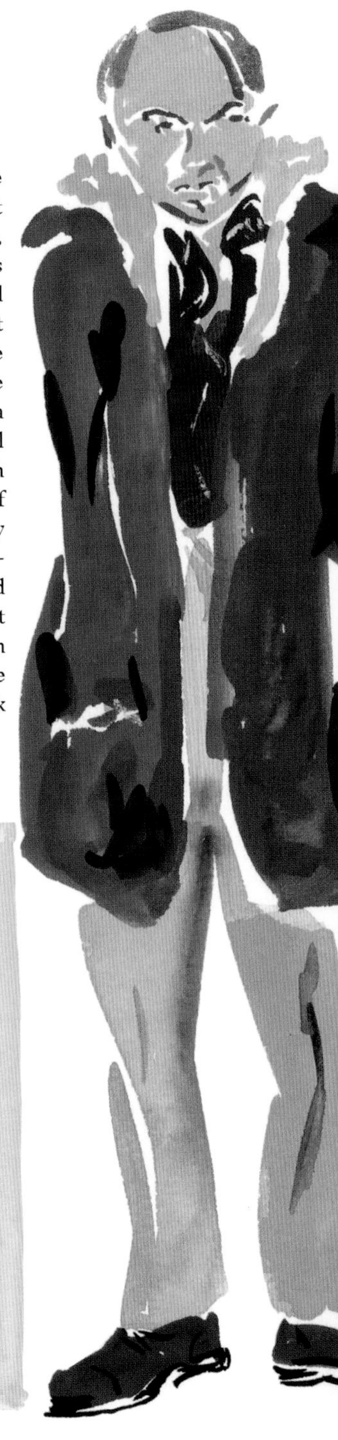

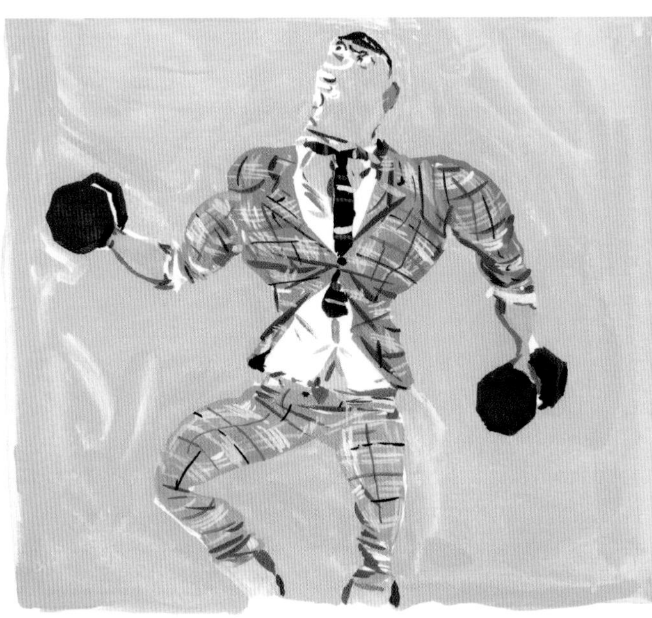

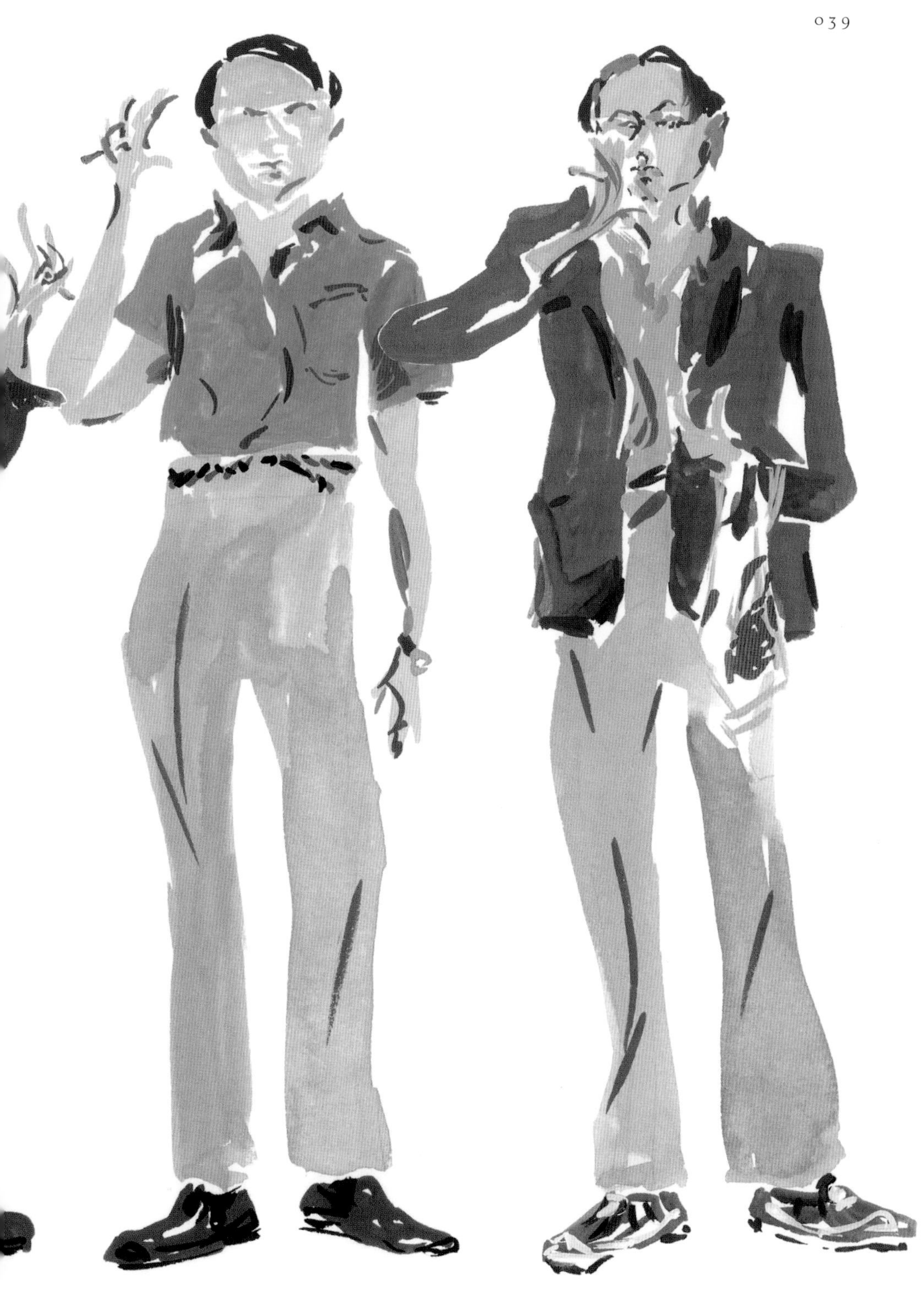

II —— 005

SHOULD YOU PICK A STRAND OF HAIR OFF SOMEONE'S SHOULDER?

Among monkeys, delousing one's peers is said to strengthen group cohesion. It is how the weakest monkeys request assistance and protection from the strongest. It is also a rather effective way for the monkey to gain popularity while serving a common cause. In both cases, the fleas are chewed up without any raised eyebrows. But trouble is on the horizon. Nothing and nobody can keep you from noticing a similarity with our venerable primate ancestors when, in the hallway, a colleague pulls a fallen hair from your shoulder. The worst thing is that he doesn't even realize he's doing it. Whatever his motives, rebuff him.

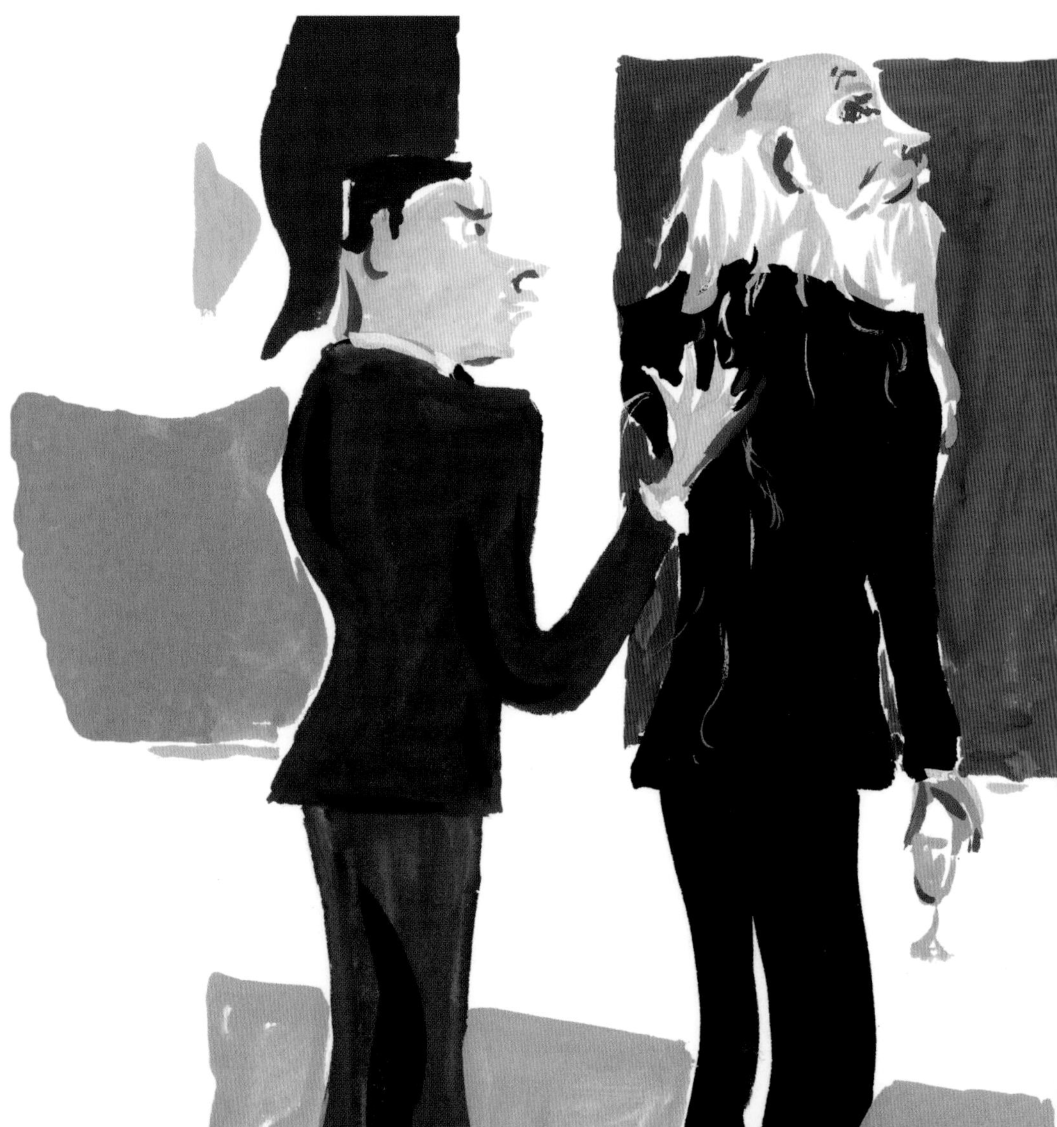

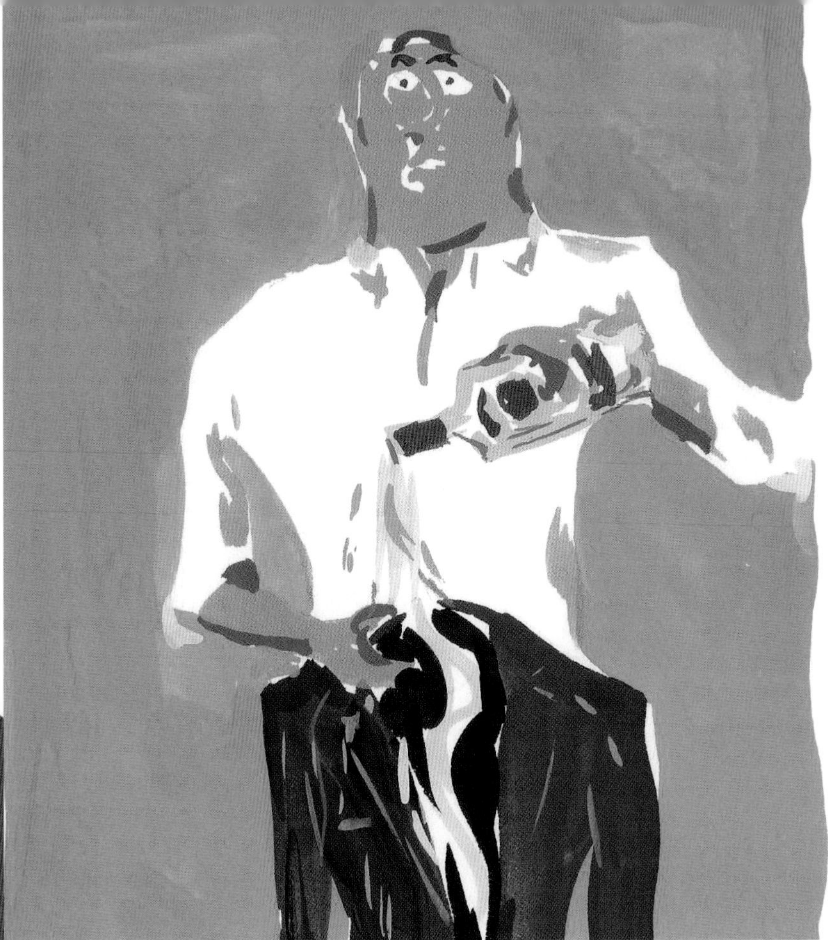

II —— 006

HOW DO YOU FRESHEN UP CLOTHES THAT REEK OF CHEESE FONDUE?

Cheese fondue: that classic dish of European ski resorts. Tempting as it is to eat, the olfactory repercussions are formidable. Besides the fuzzy tongue and cheese nightmares, you and your clothes stink. But help is at hand: before bedtime, prepare a solution of one part vodka to three parts water, and spray it abundantly on your clothes. Hang them in a well-ventilated area. The result, as you'll be astonished to discover, is tantamount to a miracle.

II —— 007

BOXERS OR BRIEFS?

The (somewhat pathetic) boxer short—if only because of its name—tries to prove it's the embodiment of potency, whereas briefs—the signature of superheroes—have no such pretensions. A pair of briefs just is. We should call them "sir." They are the companion of the regular, upright guy who stands straight and lives tall, thumbs hooked into his belt. As for the boxer, it still remains the undergarment that is best tolerated at the breakfast table.

XLII

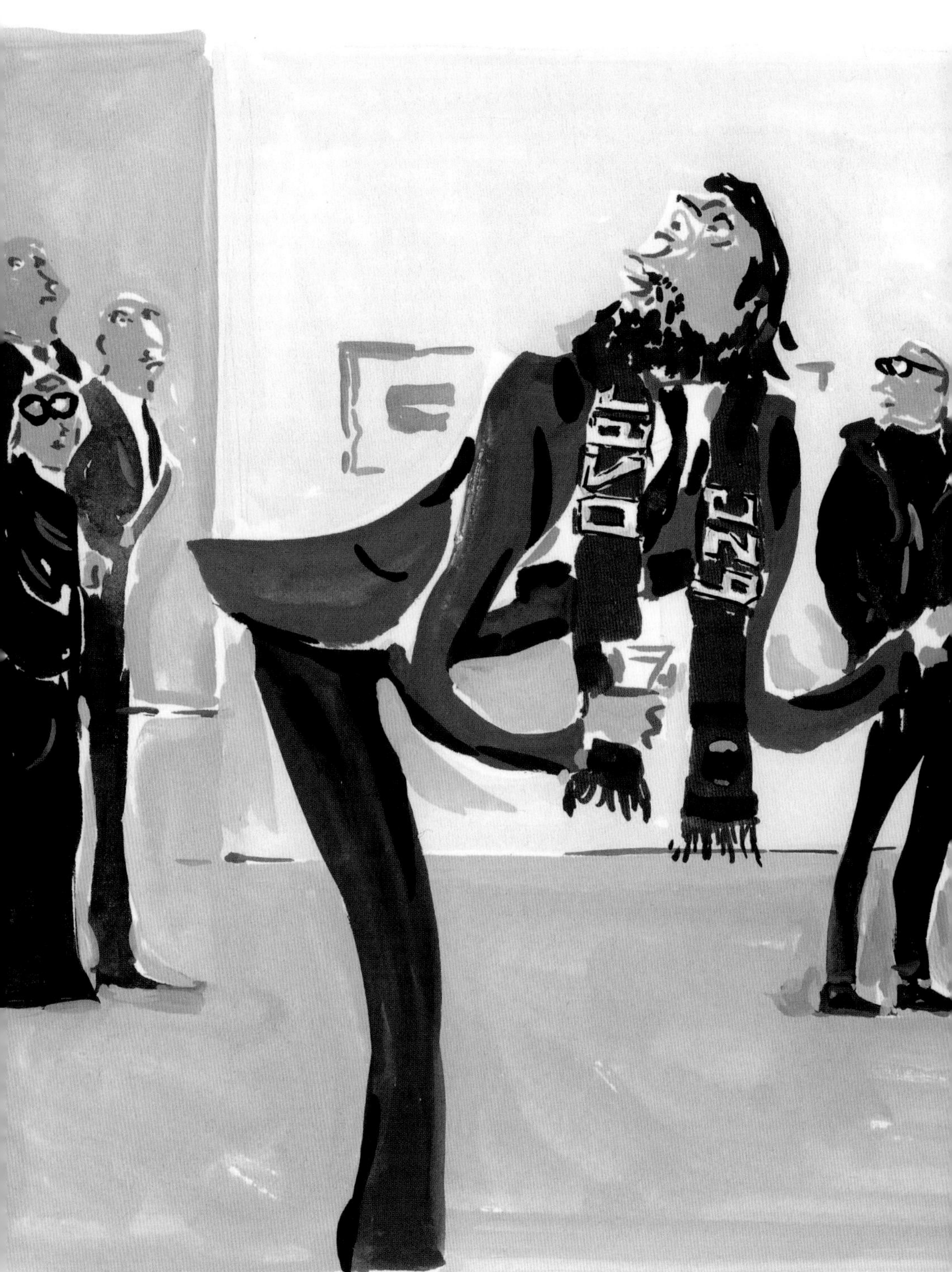

FOOL WITH THE RULES

II — 008
CAN A GENTLEMAN WEAR SPORTS PARAPHERNALIA WITH A SUIT?

Some men actually do this from time to time. The result, we must admit, is striking. It's a trick well suited to 0.001 percent of the population. And although it violates our principles, we feel like shouting it out—yes, a team scarf, outside of its context, can save an outfit. Careful, however: the irony can only work for a while. You'll soon grow tired of your little fashion combo, and you'll seek recourse in new, ever more dubious combinations. Whichever you choose, the aim is the same: to wow the observer of life who resides within you, and who sometimes turns to scrutinize himself.

II — 009
WHY IS CHIVALRY DEAD?

Because it's a major drag! Constantly paying attention to others, especially the object of one's desire, is a task that requires continuous observation and calculating everything down to the last detail.

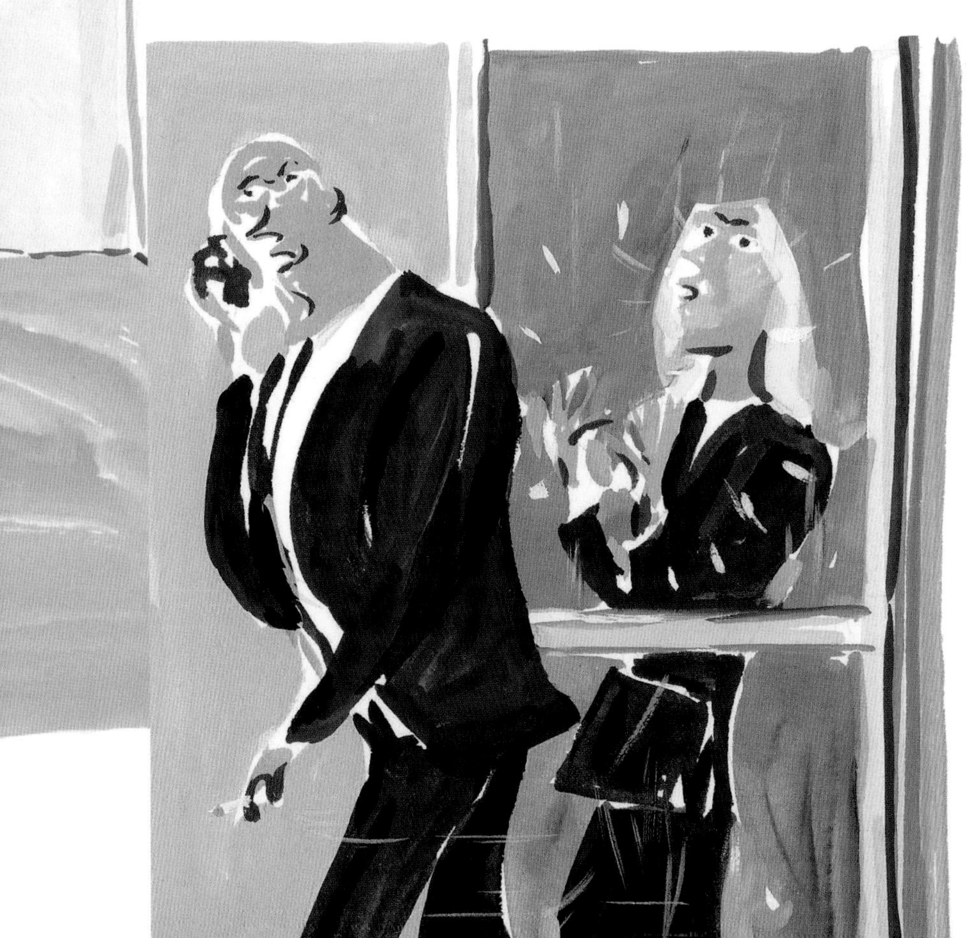

II — 010

HAVE SCALLOPS GONE FISHY?

In the 1980s, the French covered their favorite hermaphrodite—the *coquille Saint-Jacques*—in béchamel sauce, coated it with breadcrumbs, browned it in the oven, and, having reached such heavenly heights, turned the scallop shell into a pretty ashtray. The mollusk, whose beige male reproductive organ is traditionally called its "coral," used to live like a prince, riding the crest of one of Botticelli's waves. Lately, however, the scallop has lost all its charm. On our plate, its opulent coral no longer commands our attention, but has been reduced to an emulsion. As for the shell, no one wants anything to do with it anymore. Scallops have changed. They've become bourgeois. The carefree spirit of the 1980s has been forgotten, and they have become clean, organized, discreet. Whether raw or cooked, the scallop muscle governs everything from the center of the plate, lying on a bed of spinach, with a bit of coral sauce served on the side. Haughty, puritanical, trendy, pathetic—things are just not the same. Rumor has it that an official request to be rechristened Yves Saint Jacques is pending.

II — 011

At the movies, when is the right moment to plunge your hand into the popcorn?

Living your life worrying about others rarely does you any favors, but hey, why not try it once in a while? So, when you're at the movies and want to munch on popcorn, wait until the sex scene or the brawl if it's an action movie, the depressing scene in the rain if it's a French melodrama, or the stupidity-fest in a nightclub if it's an American teen comedy.

II — 012

WHAT ARE THE TEN STEPS TO NORMCORE?

The recent cult of the ordinary has a simple but rigid set of rules that anyone who grew up in the suburbs will instantly recognize. 1. Go to a hairdresser who's on the verge of bankruptcy, the kind whose display models in the window have turned yellow from the sun. 2. Hang out at a strip mall. 3. Listen to the best of Dire Straits. 4. Watch reruns of soaps and sitcoms all evening. 5. Wear high-waisted stone-washed jeans. 6. Own a limited number of socks—and only sports socks. 7. Naively believe that clothes don't make the man in a world that constantly demonstrates the opposite. 8. Wear round-toed shoes with a buckle or lace-up work boots. 9. Collect over-sized promotional T-shirts. 10. Have a penchant for frameless eyeglasses.

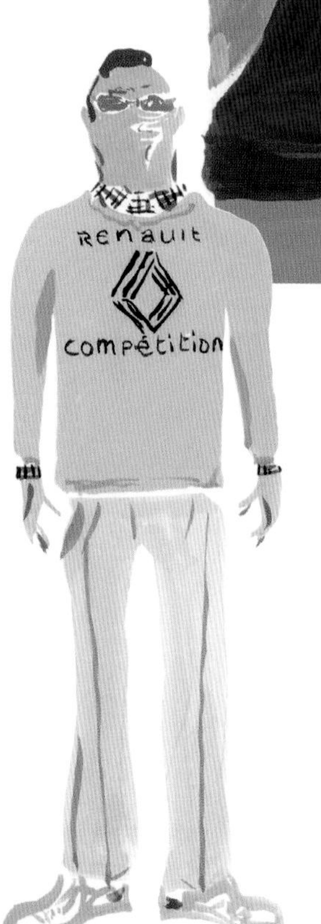

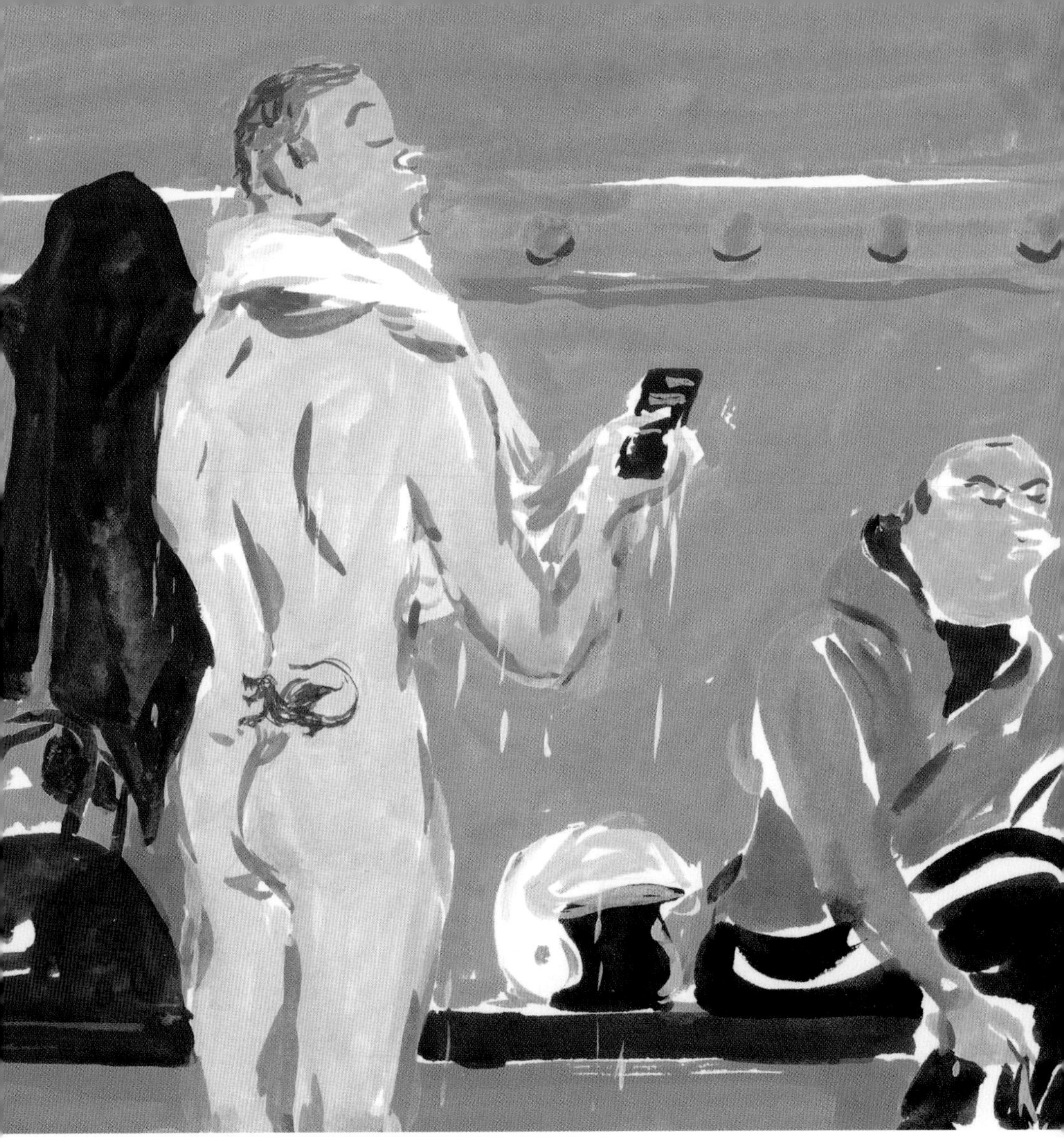

II —— 013

CAN YOU LET IT ALL HANG OUT WHEN HANGING OUT IN THE LOCKER ROOM?

Thanks to your sports savvy, your team won effortlessly. That unexpected victory has done you all a world of good. Back in the locker room with your teammates, you can revel in it. Before and after showering, you'll want to keep friendly back-slapping to a minimum while your weiner's in the open air. But in our opinion, partaking in locker-room banter shows you've got priorities that your bared privates cannot eclipse. In any form whatsoever.

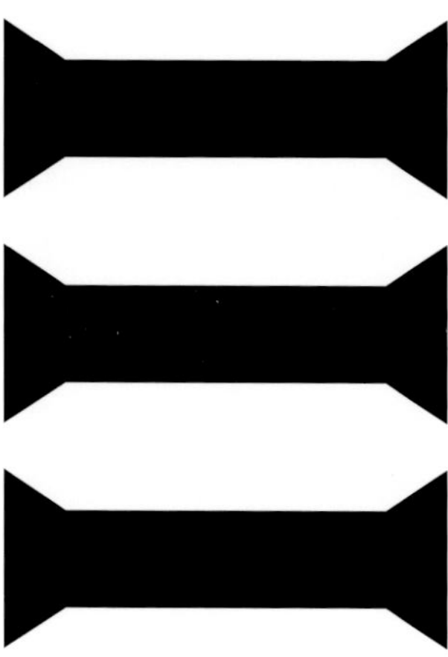

BRUSH UP ON

III —— 001 › III —— 036

How can you make an impact without even trying? • How can you act nonchalant at the vending machine? • Why do sailor T-shirts have stripes? • How should you mix prints? • How do you decode a seating plan? • What should you wear to go to vote? • What is it with the mullet? • How should you dress for air travel? • Wearing red: How can you pull it off? • How does a man in a kilt keep his socks up? • What's the point of a handkerchief? • How should you react when someone nudges your tray at the self-service counter? • Are stripes the new check? • How do you DJ with panache? • What makes a print "African-inspired"? • How can you get it right with white? • What about hand-kissing? • What should be served at a professional breakfast meeting? • Where does the

THE BASICS

polo-shirt-with-upturned-collar look come from? • Are striped T-shirts the summertime equivalent of the ski sweater? • Why is a real peacoat double-breasted? • What's the story behind the Prince of Wales check? • What can you wear with a hoodie? • How should your pant legs break over your sneakers? • Can you talk socks? • What small-town traditions make urbanites swoon? • Should you shape your beard? • How can you look suave in white at a dinner party? • The gray suit: what faux pas should you avoid? • Is it ok to layer? • How can you choose the right color socks? • Do men still do the carving these days? • To tote, or not to tote? • White jeans or colored chinos? • Are military jackets a reliable ally? • How can you spot a gentleman?

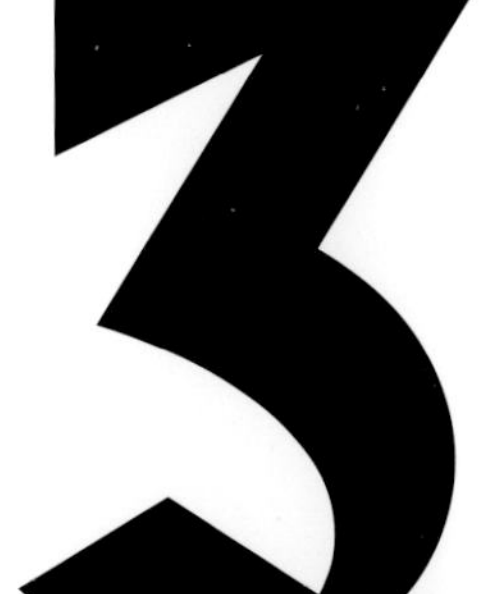

CHAPTER THREE

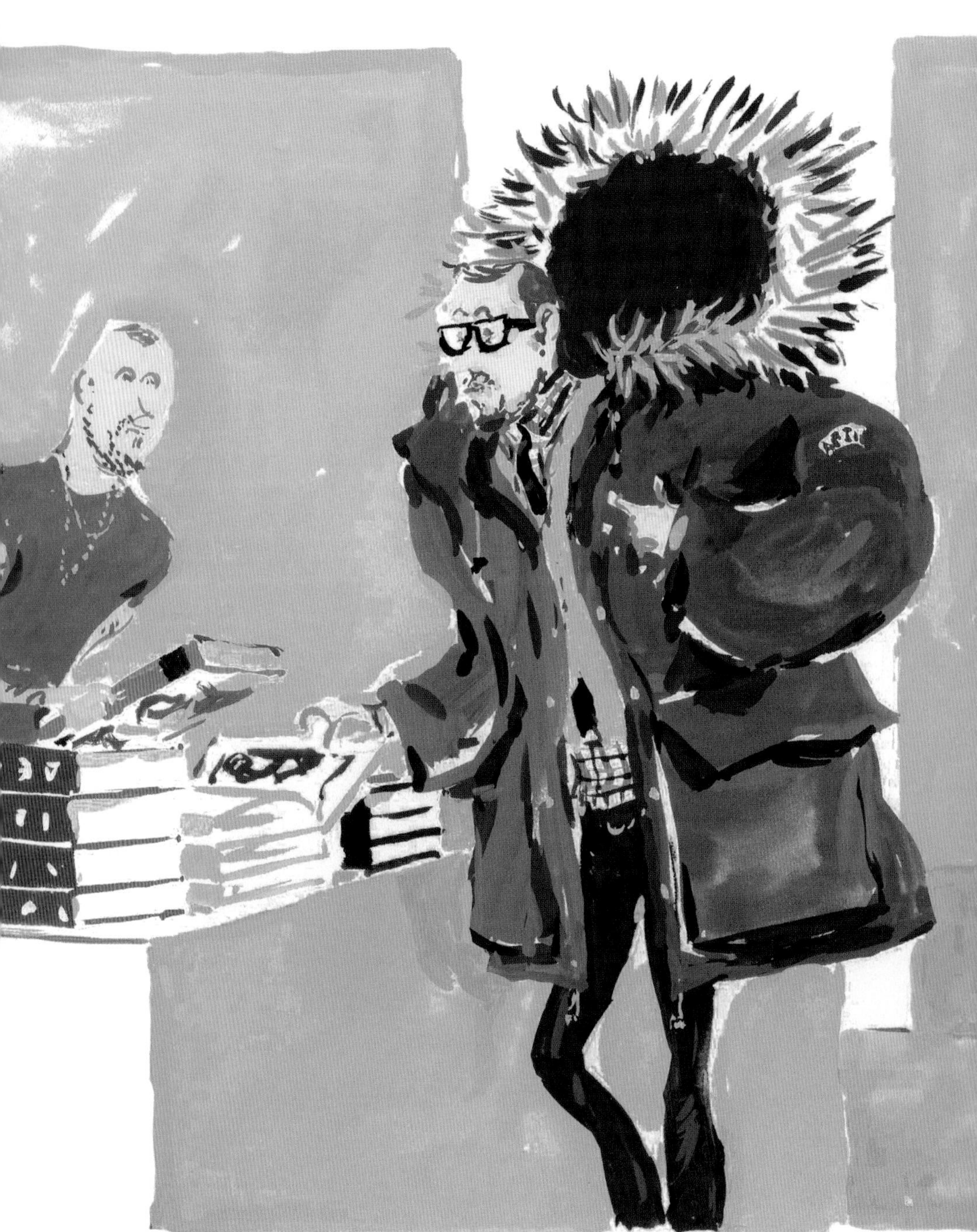

BRUSH UP ON THE BASICS

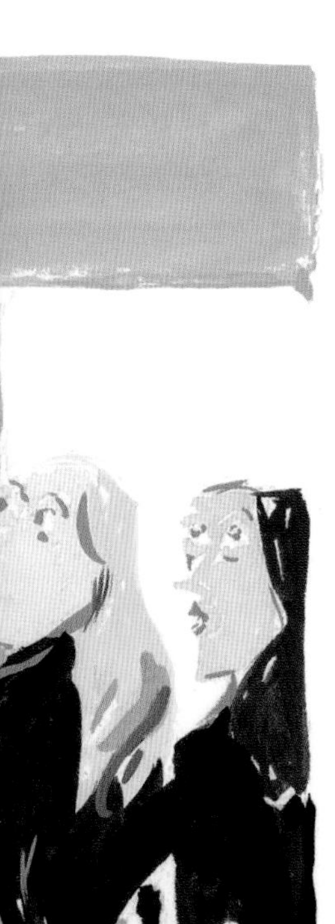

III — 001

HOW CAN YOU MAKE AN IMPACT WITHOUT EVEN TRYING?

Wearing a massive parka with the hood down in a small public space will give you instant heft. For maximum effect, you need a simple, solid-color model, either in black or khaki. A bit of a beard and a slight excess of weight will help you to impose yourself naturally in any conversation that may have started without you. Because, yes, we do expect the person who makes use of this tip to take on the role of the guy who barges right in, rather than waits around to be invited. If you get overheated and start to feel faint, unzip your coat. A word to the wise: only try this if you've already got swag and are more predator than prey.

III — 002

HOW CAN YOU ACT NONCHALANT AT THE VENDING MACHINE?

It's Monday, 6:03 pm. You decide to kill the twenty minutes separating you from freedom by heading as slowly as possible toward the vending machine. After futzing around with your change, you eventually get your candy and all is right with the world for the next three minutes. In a spontaneous gesture of lighthearted insouciance, you toss the chocolate bar into the air in front of an entire group of colleagues, who scamper away, looking busy. Unfortunately for you, the bone-tossing ape in *2001: A Space Odyssey* couldn't have done it better.

L

III —— 003

Why do sailor T-shirts have stripes?

Among other fascinating facts, Michel Pastoureau teaches us in his incredible book *L'Étoffe du diable* [The Devil's Cloth] that stripes have long stigmatized society's outcasts: acrobats, prisoners, executioners, domestics, mafiosi. Sailors are no exception. On board, their lot is not that enviable, and their military career not likely to evolve. Today, French naval officers are still called "zebras" if they are from the ranks rather than the naval college.

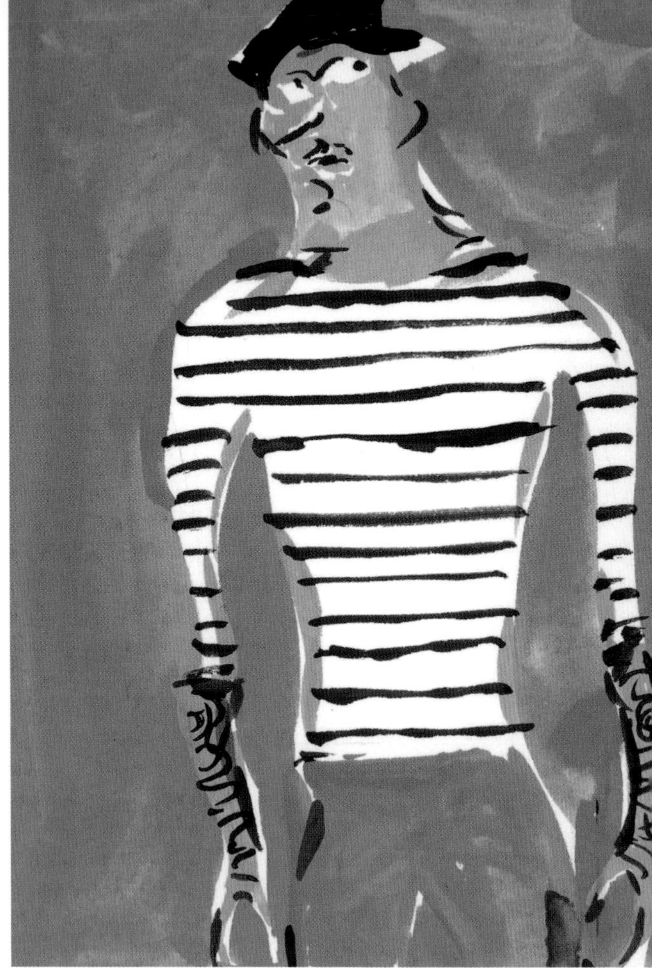

III —— 004

HOW SHOULD YOU MIX PRINTS?

The number of prints that exist is legion. Our advice: cope with the situation by gaining a little perspective. If you're wearing a pin-striped jacket with a polka-dot or paisley necktie, then stick to a solid color shirt. A pin-striped jacket and Hawaiian shirt require either a solid tie or one that doesn't stand out. Here's to fine combos!

III —— 005

HOW DO YOU DECODE A SEATING PLAN?

For those who understand how it works, table seating reveals the role you play in the lives of others. Generally speaking, guests of honor are placed on either side of the hosts and at a distance from their spouse, adversaries, and frenemies. Life-of-the-party types are sacrificed to the dull people, who are thus delightfully entertained all evening.

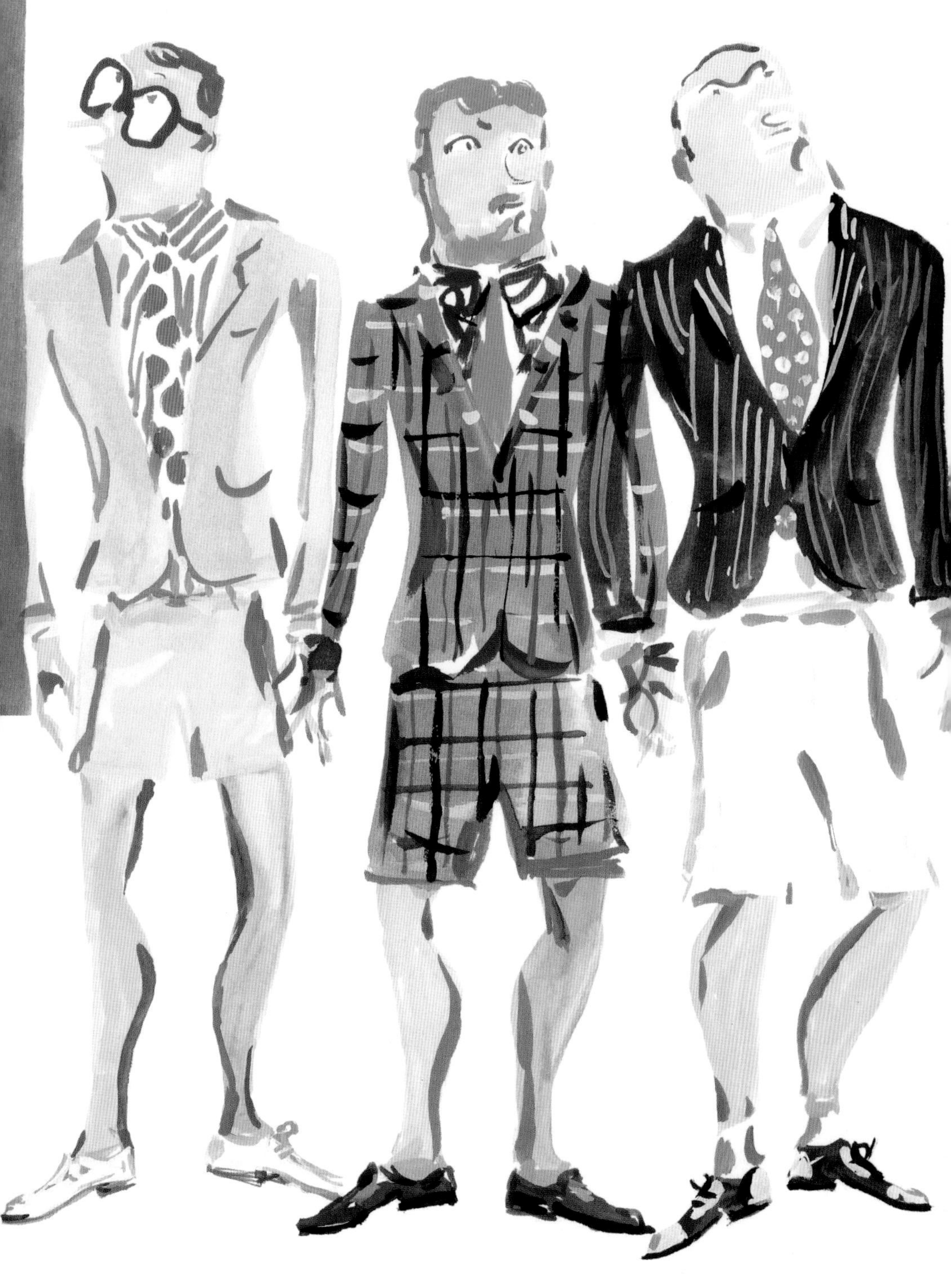

III —— 006

WHAT SHOULD YOU WEAR TO GO TO VOTE?

Since wearing distinctive political insignia is prohibited in many polling places, you'd do best not to reveal your political opinions when you go to vote (leave the T-shirts, rosettes, and partisan pins at home). After breakfast on Election Day, you'll have two possibilities: 1. Don't go and vote, in which case you'll do the dishes as you grumble about loud-mouthed, dishonest politicians. Enough said. 2. Head to the elementary school that's been turned into a political outpost. For this, we suggest a casual nondescript look—i.e., faded jeans, a white button-down or immaculate polo shirt, a pair of Chucks or desert boots, and a zip-front jacket, beige or blue parka, or, if it's drizzling out, a peacoat. Simplicity is appropriate for the seriousness of the occasion.

III —— 007

WHAT IS IT WITH THE MULLET?

Presumably some guys think it's attractive, right? And they're clinging on to memories of their heyday. Or else they're very impressed by Native American culture. Or maybe in homage to David Bowie in his Ziggy Stardust period. If you believe the official line, the advantage of the cut—short on top, long at the neck—is that it's "Business in the front, party in the back." Now it's taboo, we can't imagine what it will look like next time around. It's up to the English to decide. They're experts in this kind of thing.

III —— 008

HOW SHOULD YOU DRESS FOR AIR TRAVEL?

Far be it from us to accuse low-cost airlines of downgrading the airport dress code. That's not our style. It hasn't escaped our notice, though, that as you were preparing for your departure, you remembered to grab your passport and to resist the giant bar of Toblerone—congratulations—but it never occurred to you, even for a moment, to mark the occasion by wearing the appropriate clothes. When you fly, give wings to your wardrobe. Take a stab at creativity, by all means, but the classic combo of trousers, shirt, and jacket is good, too. And do keep comfort in mind—anyone who has experienced the horror of a long-haul flight in skinny jeans or tight shoes knows the humiliation of being eyed by the entire crew when you reach your destination.

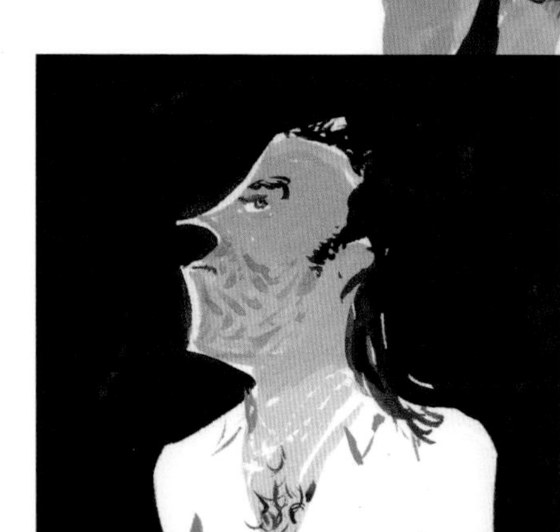

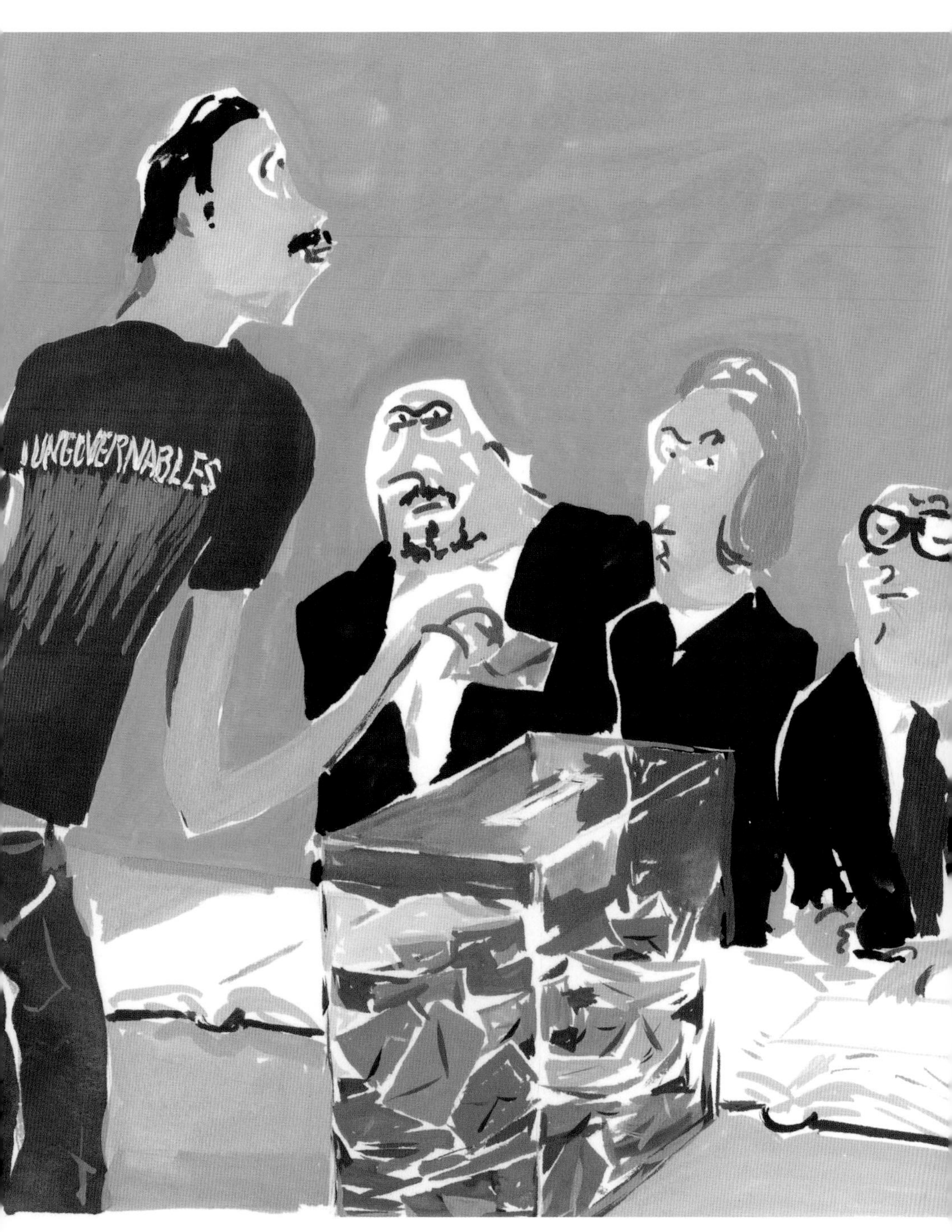
UNGOVERNABLES

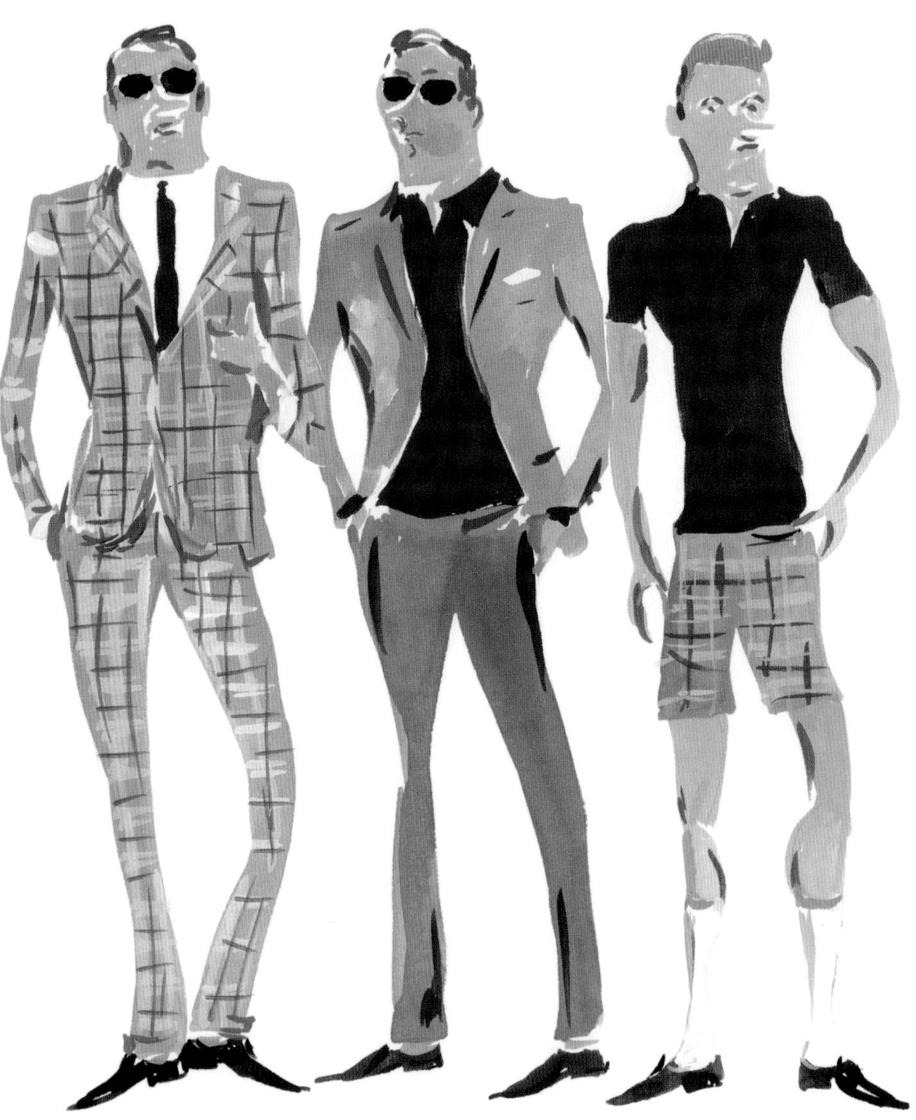

III —— 009

WEARING RED: HOW CAN YOU PULL IT OFF?

Jean-Paul Belmondo, or rather Jean-Luc Godard, helps us answer this question in *Pierrot le Fou* (1965). In the film, red plays a crucial role. It depicts violence and passion, in contrast to an omnipresent blue. The actors' costumes are pretty effective and can be summed up in two summer outfits: one is a light-gray, glen plaid suit, white shirt, red tie, and black shoes; the other is a slightly mismatched light-gray jacket and pants, with a red-pepper-colored shirt and no tie. In short, imagine yourself in charge of paprika in a hotel kitchen: dose it carefully.

III — 010

HOW DOES A MAN IN A KILT KEEP HIS SOCKS UP?

Sorry to shake up your beliefs and shatter your illusions, but there's no miracle. To hang in there all evening, drinking and dancing to the bagpipe groove, Scots pull their socks up to the knee, and then tie a garter at the top of the calf. The whole device is hidden by the sock's ribbed cuff folded down over the elastic band. This method is also used by other peoples accustomed to wearing skimpy outfits in hostile environments—hence our Scottish example, but it is equally pertinent in Austria. Under the pleated skirt that you might someday sport, wear boxers or, like a true Scot, nothing at all. Whatever your choice, do not give in to the questions of the curious-minded. No matter how insistent their whiskey-fueled inquiries become, keep this information to yourself. Defend your honor like Mel Gibson in *Braveheart*.

III — 011

What's the point of a handkerchief?

A pocket square by default, a handkerchief enables you not only to wipe your brow between two waltzes (out of breath, eh?), but also to clean the screen of your cell phone or any other portable device.

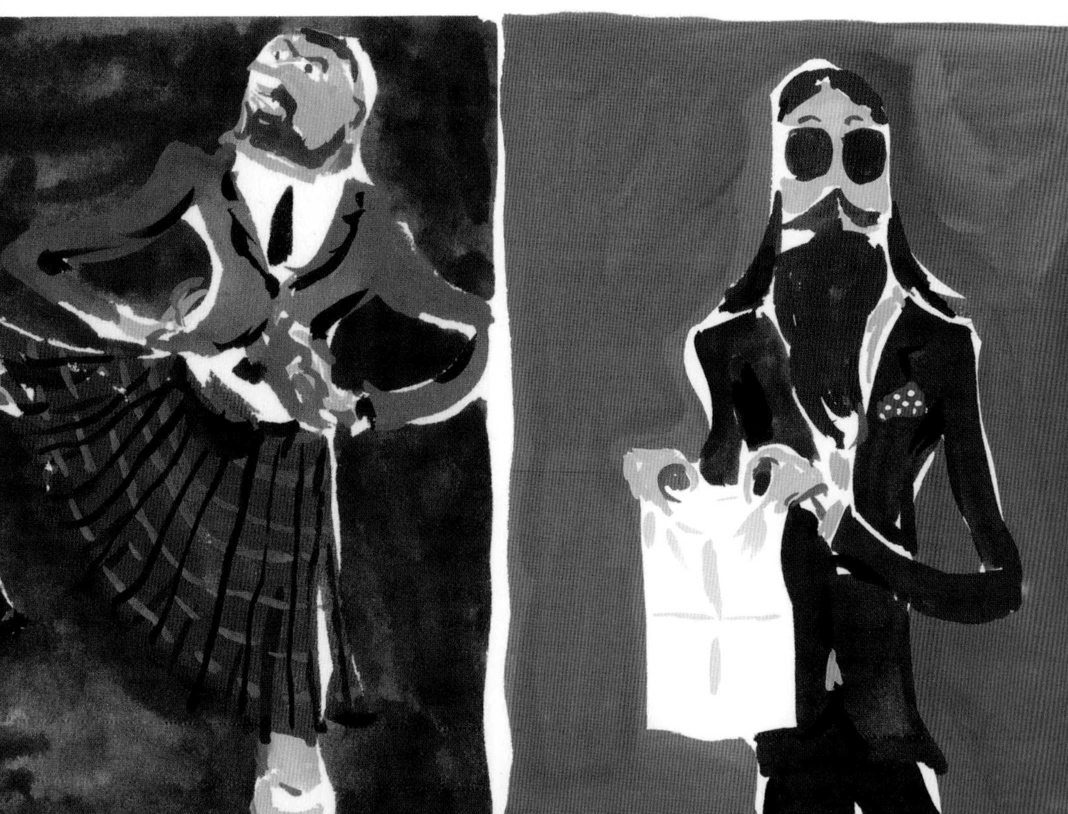

III —— 012

HOW SHOULD YOU REACT WHEN SOMEONE NUDGES YOUR TRAY AT THE SELF-SERVICE COUNTER?

As you are retrieving your plate of macaroni and cheese, your tray appears to shoot forward of its own volition. The person behind this outrage has, in fact, quite enough space to wait his turn. Maintaining superhuman levels of *sangfroid,* you cast an icy look in the knucklehead's direction in retaliation. Shaken up by such a display of self-control, he will doubtless have to go on sick leave, which, one can only hope, will teach him to improve his cafeteria line behavior in the future.

III —— 013

Are stripes the new check?

We are noting a marked return to stripes, which will certainly please you. Always go for thin over thick and vertical over horizontal stripes (unless you are wearing a sailor T-shirt, of course). Black, blue, green, and red stripes are allowed. It's as simple as that. Very important: the lightest color should always be the dominant one.

III —— 014

HOW DO YOU DJ WITH PANACHE?

Since every Tom, Dick, and Harry knows how to line up one hit song after another, dealing with this essential question seemed important to us. Get rid of the headset: it serves no purpose. Playing with the bass, medium, and treble levels is all a matter of dosage. Focus on the bass sounds when they get louder. Mute them, then fling them back in for the drop. Sometimes it's tough getting the party started: the crowd stands there, backlit, eyes glued to their screens. So just keep smiling and look focused so no one comes to steal your place and put Abba back on. P.S.: Before whipping out your bad-boy tunes, get the girls on your side. Otherwise you're screwed.

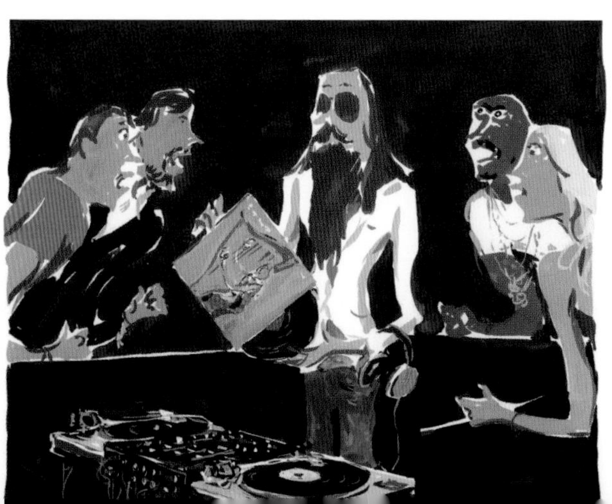

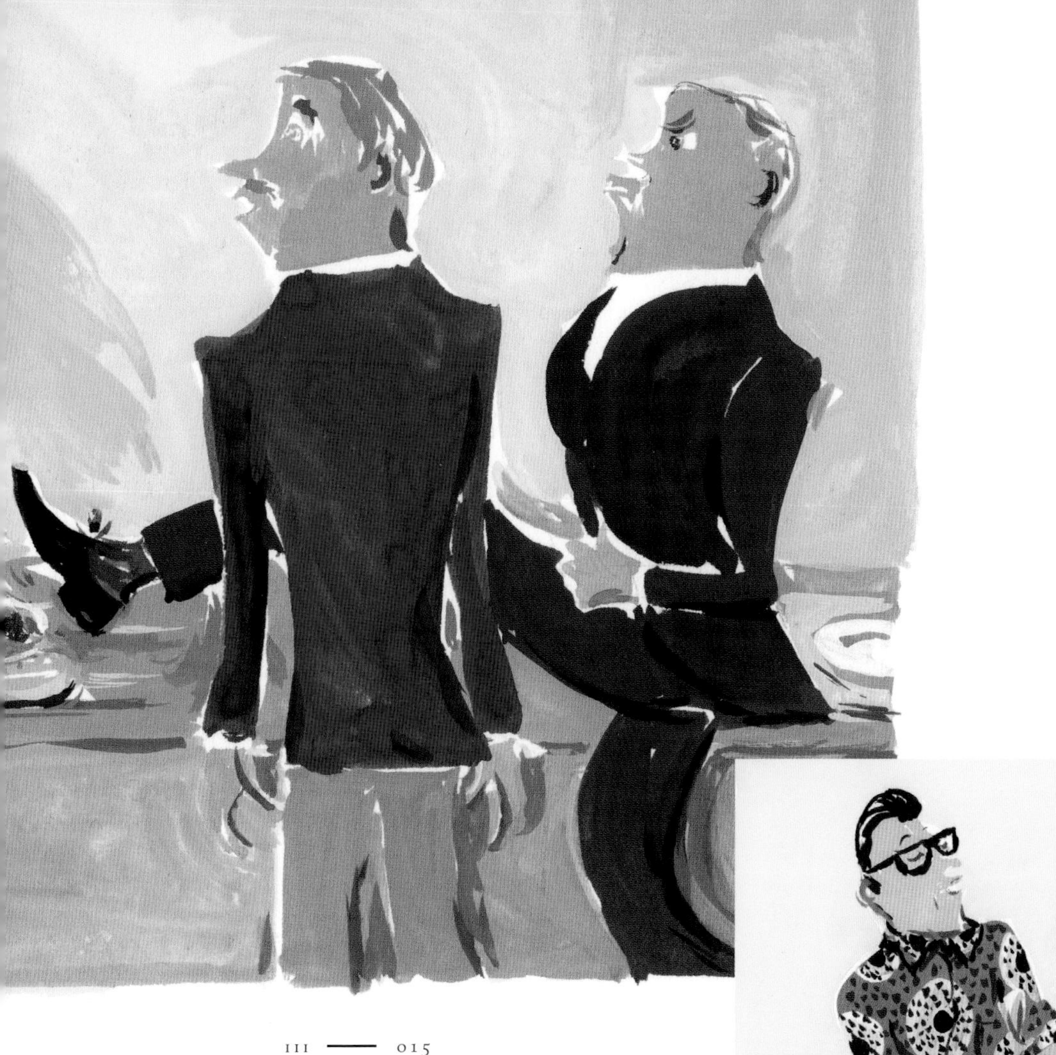

III —— 015

WHAT MAKES A PRINT "AFRICAN-INSPIRED"?

The term "African-inspired," or even just "African," is often bandied about when it comes to prints, whether rightly or wrongly, because current trends celebrate the continent that cradled humanity. Generally speaking, if the pattern makes you blink, it's considered of African inspiration. The color contrasts are strong and the patterns original: lots of geometric shapes, shells, abstract designs, and very warm colors. Everything glows and radiates. Often the prints are full-on psychedelic. Keep a cool head and choose what you like, not just what's in fashion. Don't stand out from the crowd for the wrong reasons.

III —— 016

HOW CAN YOU GET IT RIGHT WITH WHITE?

A little reminder of items that work: 1. Whiter than white: a T-shirt or undershirt, perfect when tucked into dark chinos or black jeans. For optimum results, we recommend watching your waistline. Slim-fit jeans, worn with a pale button-down shirt and dark blazer, for the classic Swinging London look. A button-down shirt that will follow you into the grave. A polo shirt that will always have your back. A pair of briefs: a man's best friend. 2. Clever white: tending toward blue, gray, or ivory to tone it down. Perfect for a cotton or linen-blend suit or for giving more depth to a fisherman's sweater or pair of pants. 3. Dirty white: shoes or sneakers, in buckskin or canvas. They've taken quite a beating from kicking those cans around, and are all the better for it.

III —— 017

What about hand-kissing?

According to French etiquette, the custom of bowing and lightly touching a proffered hand with your lips is never to be practiced in public places or out in the open. Hands must be bare, and the circumstances appropriate. It is a courtesy reserved for married women. Unless you're something of a scamp.

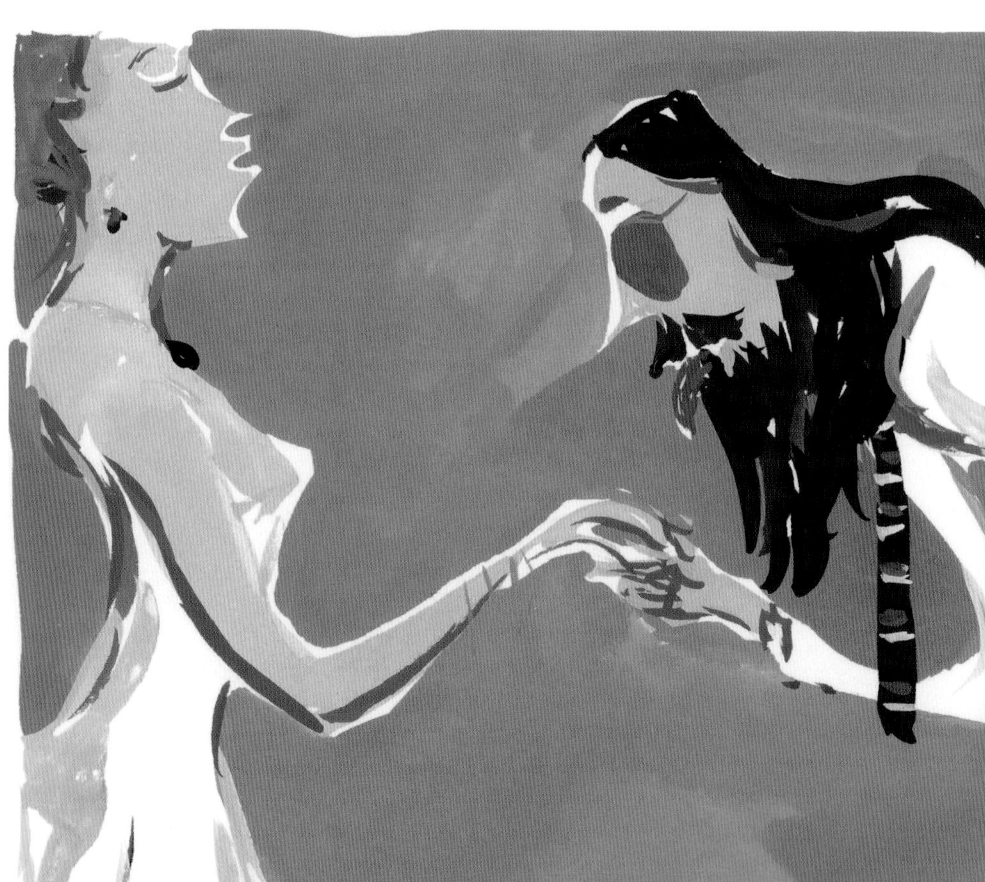

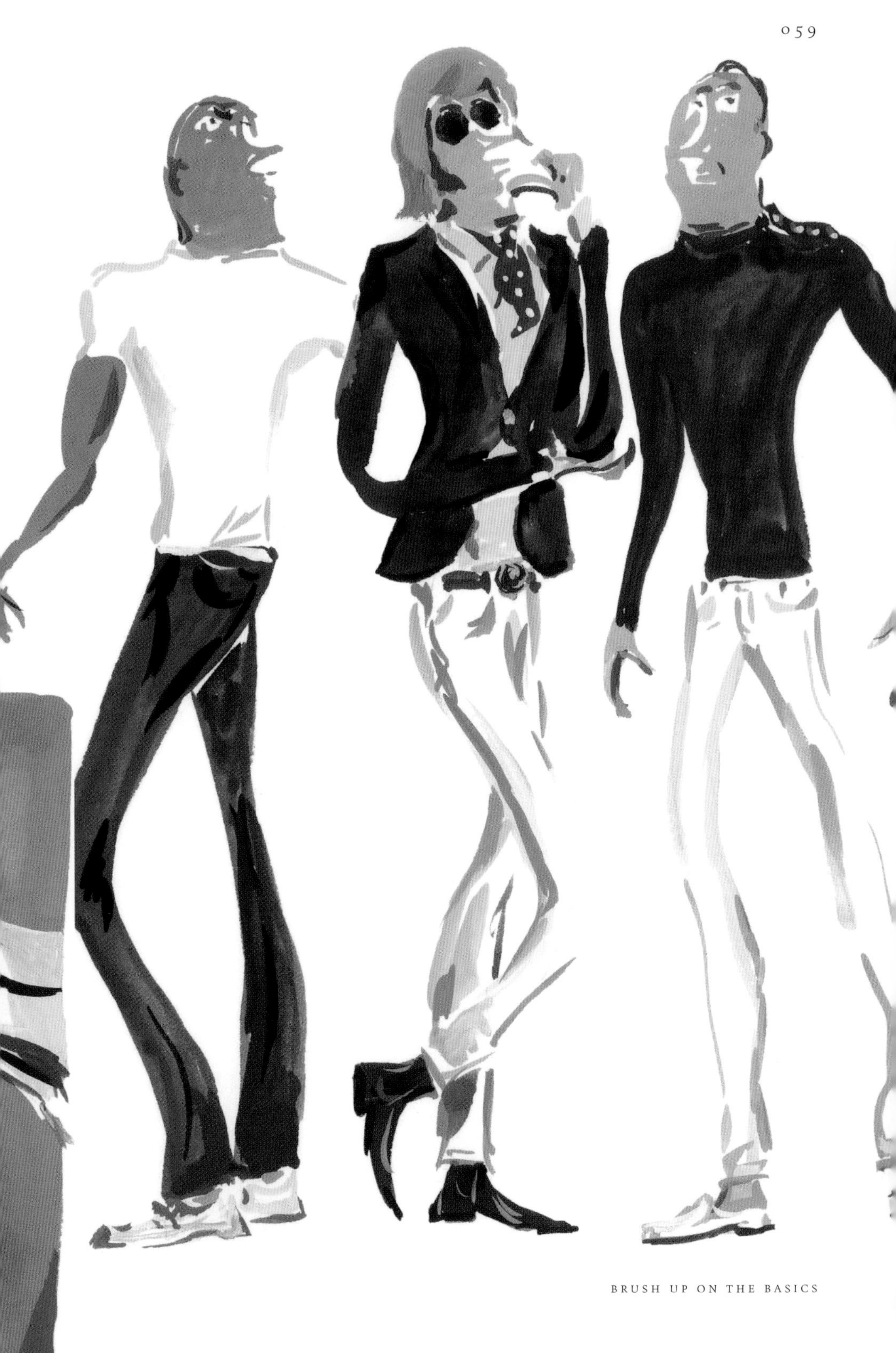

III —— 018

WHAT SHOULD BE SERVED AT A PROFESSIONAL BREAKFAST MEETING?

One fine morning, the boss calls in the entire staff for a breakfast meeting of champions, to reveal the major points of the company's new strategy. The pastries on the table are a reflection of the firm's future. With the amount of mini-croissant crumbs left under the chairs, you could create a flowchart on messiness. Horrified, you convert to donuts.

III —— 019

Where does the polo-shirt-with-upturned-collar look come from?

From a business school somewhere in hell. Or from the great English upper class, which, with a mere sweep of the hand, repeatedly humiliates its adversaries at polo. Or from the desire to be immortal, seated on the right-hand side of soccer player Eric Cantona. In short, much like a peacock proudly displaying its tail feathers, this look stems from the urge to intimidate a rival group.

III —— 020

ARE STRIPED T-SHIRTS THE SUMMERTIME EQUIVALENT OF THE SKI SWEATER?

Previously, on the slopes in your awful ski sweater, you looked at best like a huge snowflake. Now the air is warm again and the sea beckons. You want the sailor look. Please note that we vastly prefer this striped model to its mountaintop counterpart.

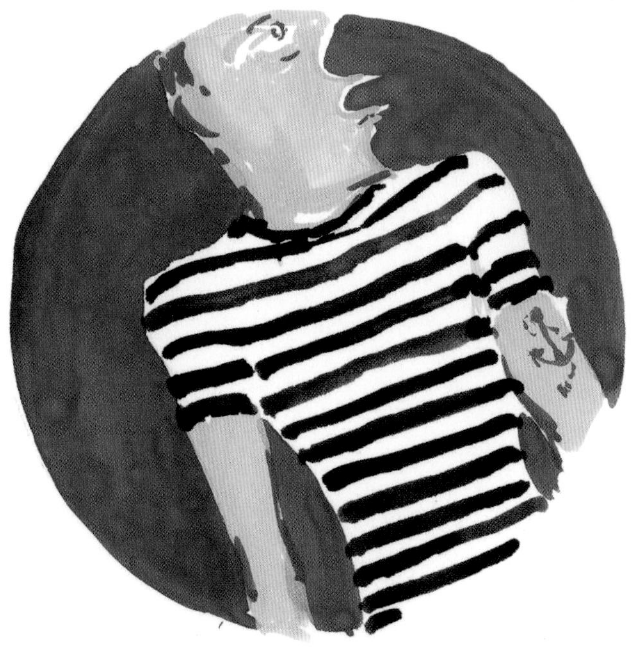

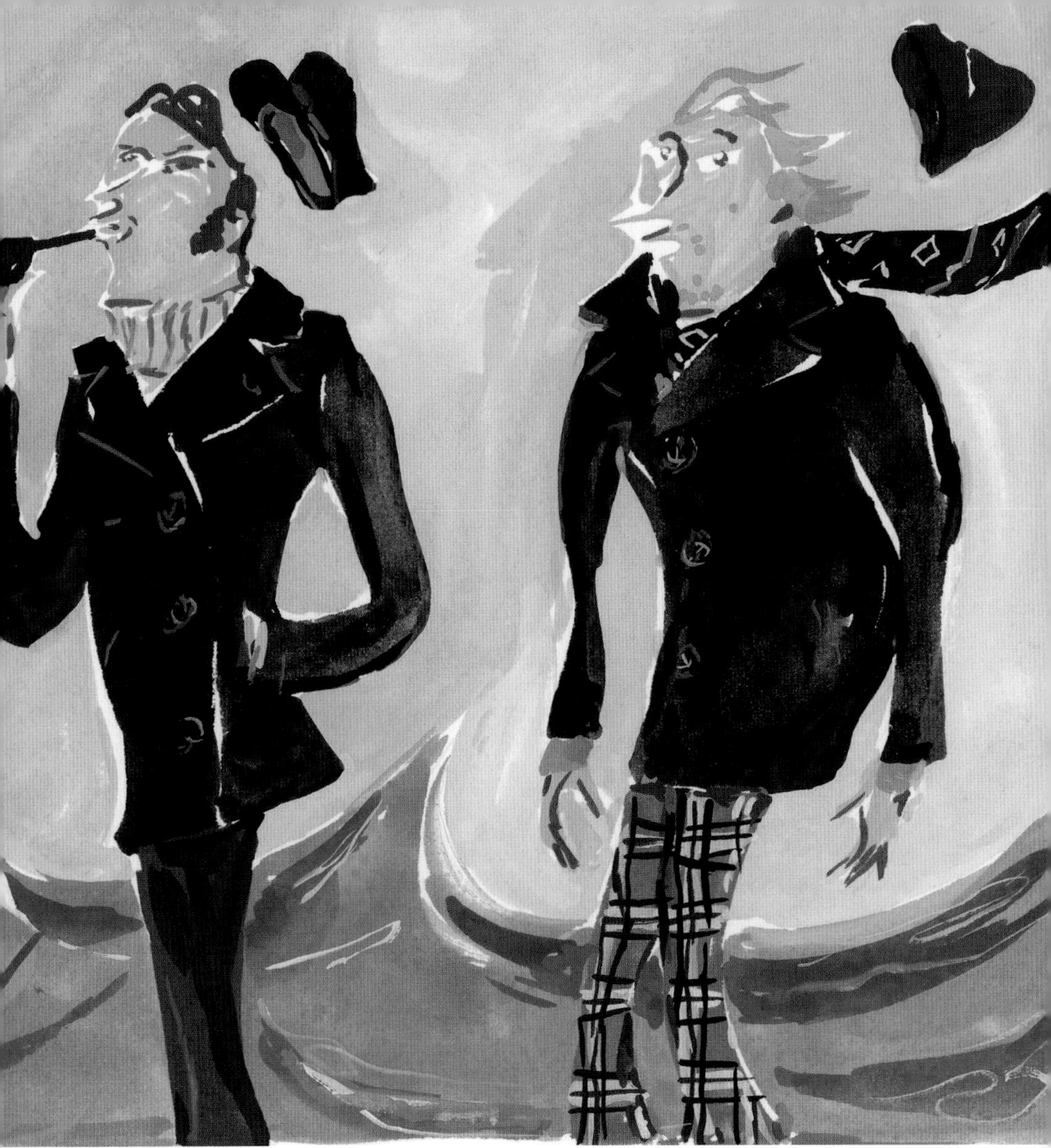

III —— 021

WHY IS A REAL PEACOAT DOUBLE-BREASTED?

This is no small matter. Take a minute to think about how having buttoning options might stylishly improve your next trip to the coast. Imagine yourself for a moment facing the wind, rocked by the waves. What unfortunate mishap could befall you? By what means might you risk losing, in a split second, your dignity and standing? You're almost there. The answer to our question? The peacoat can be buttoned up on either side because the side facing the wind should cover the other. That way your garment won't fill up with air. Lifesaving.

LXII

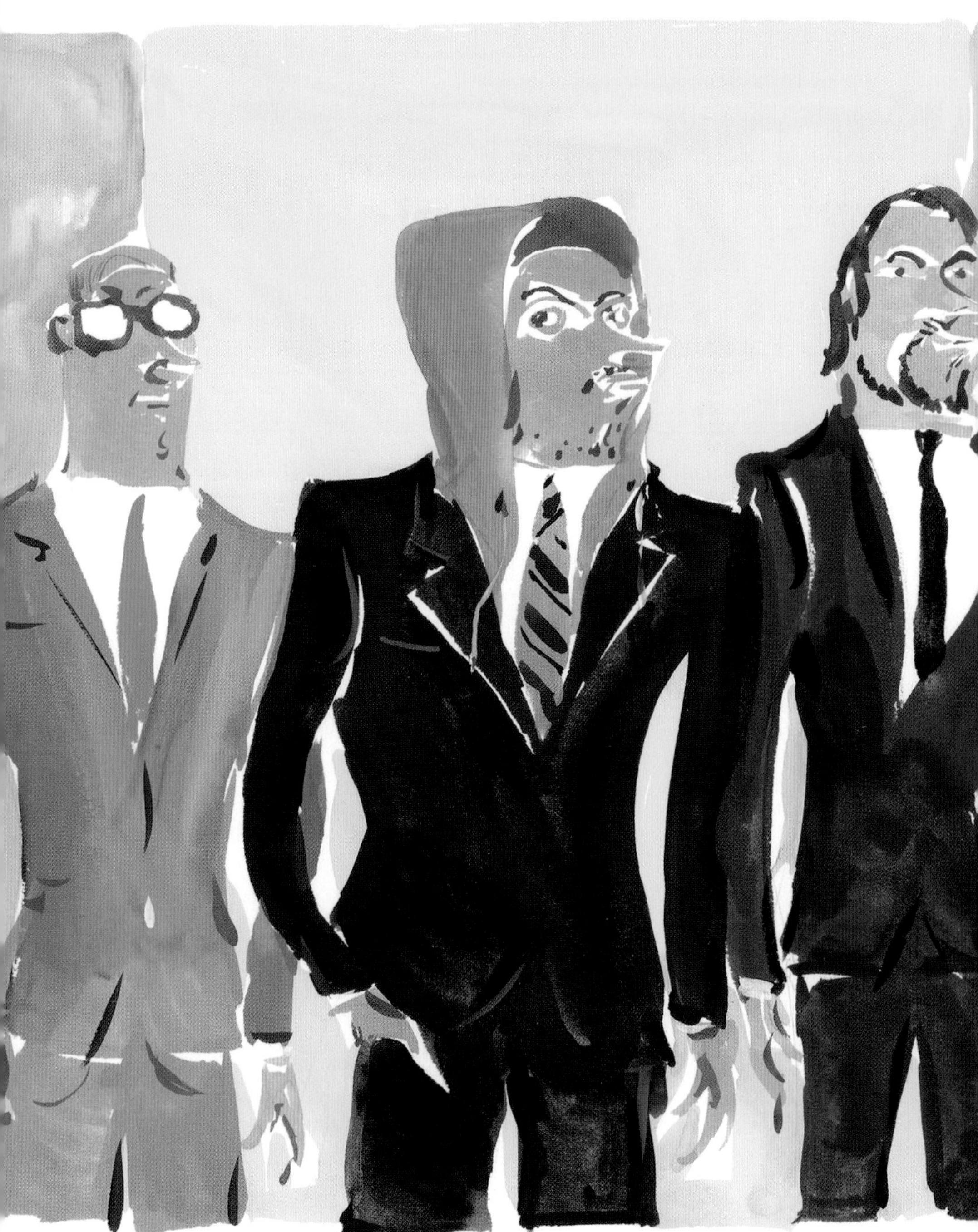

BRUSH UP ON THE BASICS

III — 022

WHAT'S THE STORY BEHIND THE PRINCE OF WALES CHECK?

Edward, Prince of Wales and future king of England, was called the "king of fashion." On weekends he liked to go hunting in Scotland, a rather posh destination back then. Being a fashion victim, he wasn't immune to the charms of the tartans the local clans wore—the equivalent of familial coats of arms. In keeping with custom, those who do not belong to any clan but possess an estate may wear a humble "district check," allowing them to partake of a little local color. In Glenurquhart, Inverness-shire, the glen plaid is worn. When Edward arrived, he shot everything that moved on the Mar estate. There he wore a variation of the glen plaid with blue stripes named after the estate. He later perfected the plaid and exported it to the rest of the world as soon as he ascended to the throne of England in 1901.

III — 023

What can you wear with a hoodie?

Between seasons, you have to make a choice, but you can do so without looking like an idiot. In springtime, it's all about layering because it's too warm, or too cool, or too unpredictable. With that in mind, the hoodie, or hooded sweatshirt, offers dual benefits: the hood keeps the cold and humidity out, while you can tie it around your waist if it's too warm. We all agree that wearing a hoodie with nothing else looks stupid. And it doesn't work with your office coat, a blazer, or a velvet jacket. However, overcoats, bomber jackets, and military and workmen's jackets are all good.

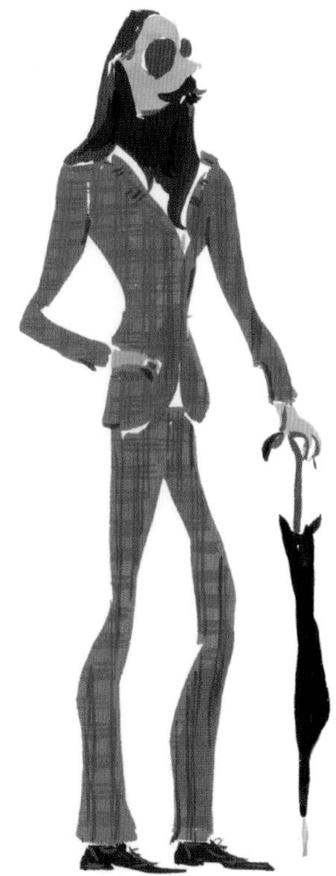

III —— 024

HOW SHOULD YOUR PANT LEGS BREAK OVER YOUR SNEAKERS?

The question is simpler than it seems. Whether your sneakers are high or low is up to you. But if you wear the kind of oldies that are clean, simple, and poorly suited to playing sports (Converse, Stan Smith, Cortez, etc.), then you'll wear them like classic city shoes, meaning with pants slightly rolled up at the ankles. For kids who owe their existence to 1980s technology and design, and are wedded to the hightop (from the Air Max 90 to LeBron James models), the rule dictates that the hem of your pants be unrolled until it breaks two or three times. Watch out, though, for the accordion that appears when the surplus fabric bunches up and falls onto the tongue of the shoe. When in socks, your heel should be stepping on the hem of your pants.

III —— 025

Can you talk socks?

Now that you've become a fashion geek, you can enjoy memorizing the anatomy of the sock. You'll see, it's fascinating. You'll learn to locate the cuff, leg (easy), instep, gusset, heel flap, heel turn, sole, and the toe. Bravo, Bobby.

III —— 026

WHAT SMALL-TOWN TRADITIONS MAKE URBANITES SWOON?

Coveralls that are no big deal in the boonies become the latest must-have in cosmopolitan cities. Remember that hotdog stand on the beach, where no gulls or bathers hung out—the one that smelled like grease and ketchup? Transfer it to Paris and it becomes a food truck, the hip new fast-food service for office workers in the know. There used to be a van that went around rural France on Sundays, stopping in small-town squares and residential areas, selling tools and clothes and whatnot. Would you believe there's a new variation of it? The fashion truck! The truck parks next to skyscrapers in the city so that the business-suited, capitalist proletariat—never mind the words, comrade—can, in the time it takes to have lunch, have tailored suits made at market prices.

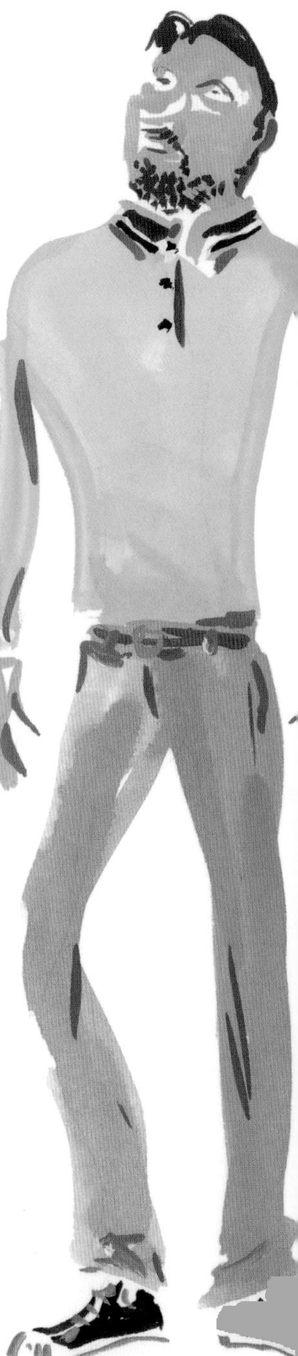

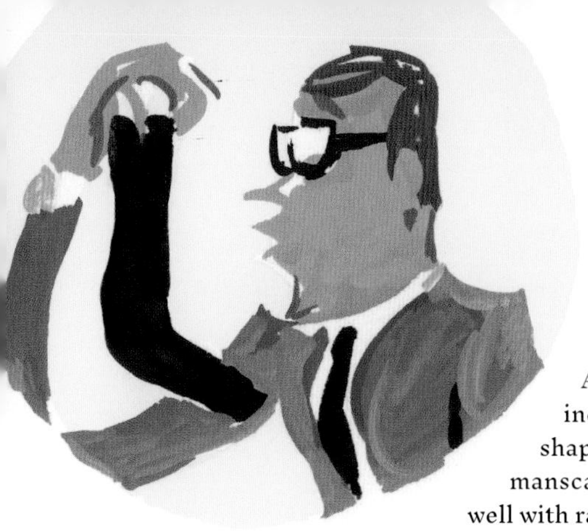

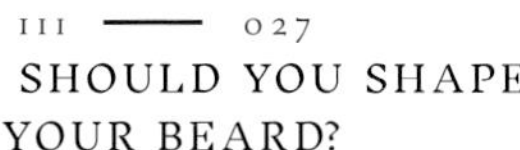

III — 027

SHOULD YOU SHAPE YOUR BEARD?

As you will have noticed, some ill-advised individuals go to unreasonable lengths to shape their beard. This is just the tip of the manscaping iceberg. A designer beard works well with rap artists who don't want to look like Isaac Hayes, but guys hoping for street cred by borrowing the technique from their streetwise brothers will immediately be reduced to the status of Ken—and we don't mean the Survivor: we're talking Barbie dolls here. Um, no, this is not a compliment. If your idea of adventure is shaping your facial hair, think about getting a close shave. This simple gesture will be the wisest move in tough times.

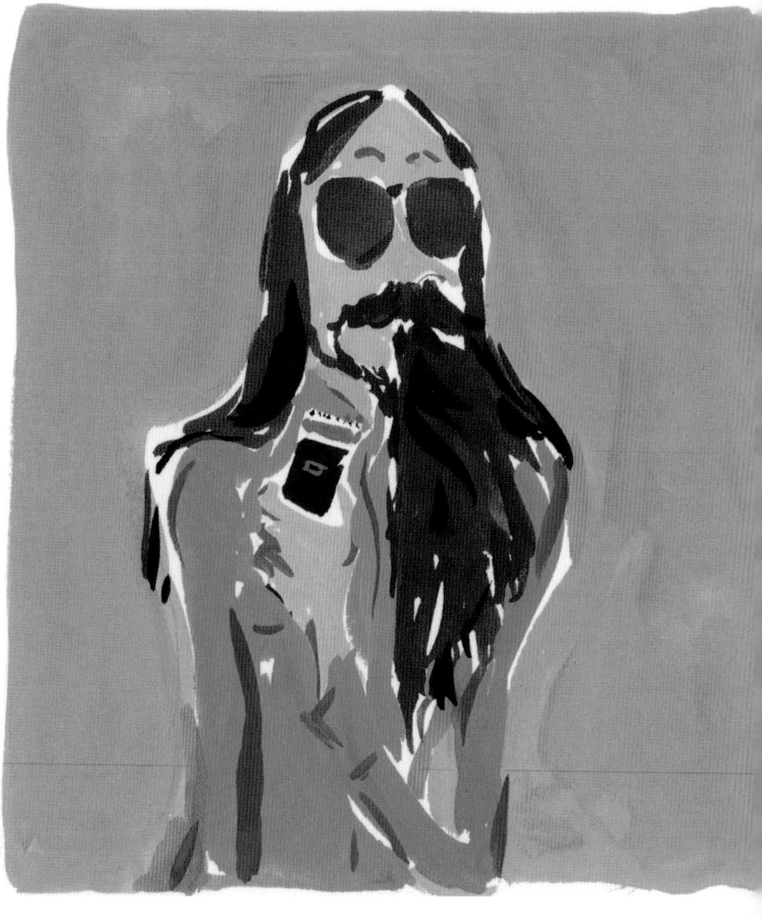

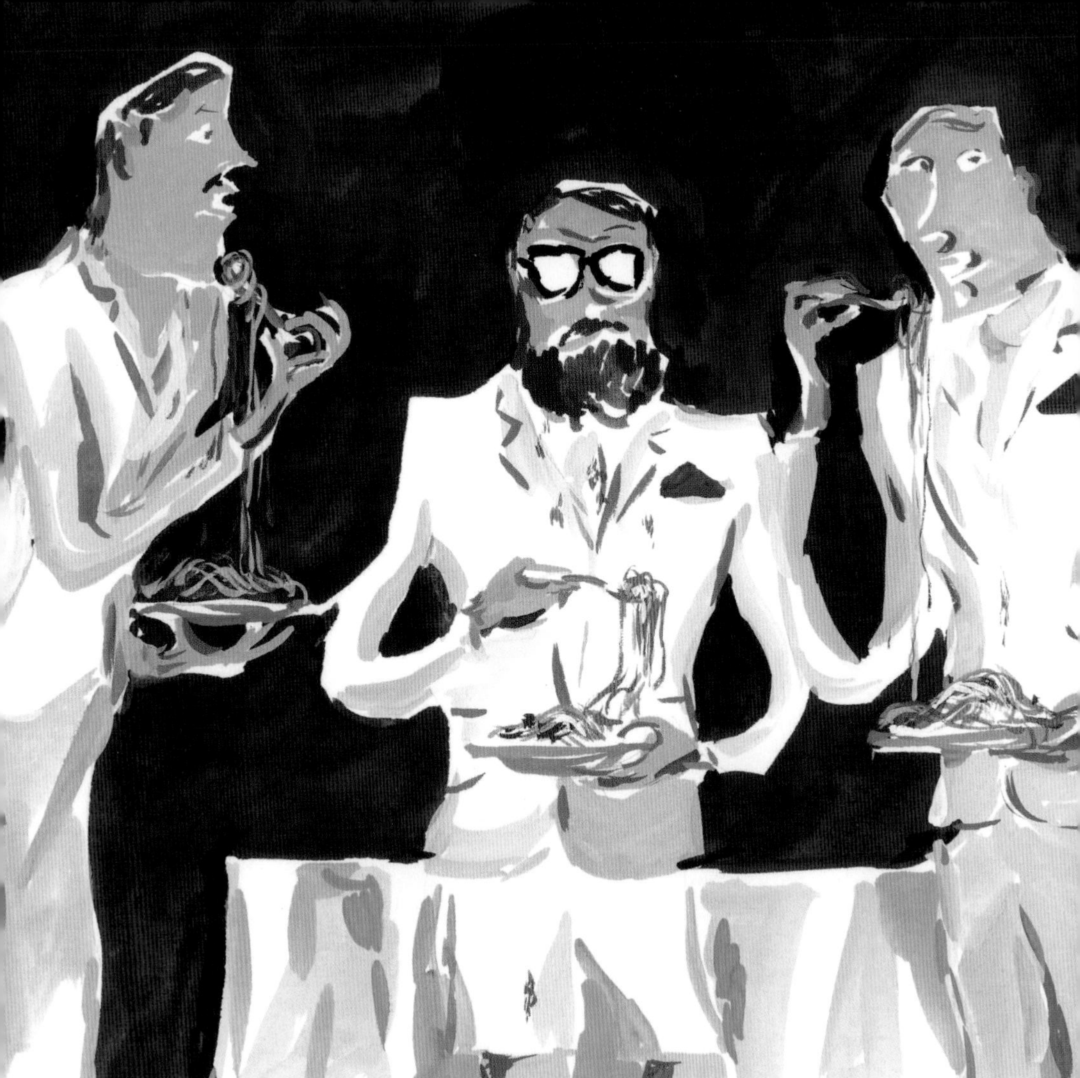

III —— 028

HOW CAN YOU LOOK SUAVE IN WHITE AT A DINNER PARTY?

One of your colleagues has the crazy idea of choosing a "white" theme for his birthday dinner. So now you're worried about looking like a nurse, baker, tennis player, or Liberace. Instead, take a leaf out of writer Tom Wolfe's book. With him, sometimes the white becomes cream, and is even more flamboyant when there's a dash of color to heighten it, like a sky-blue shirt and a black tie and shoes. You can invest in white jeans, chinos, or Bermudas; white sneakers with colorful details; and a white shirt or polo shirt. Add a light-gray or pastel cardigan or jacket, and you're all set. It's the spirit that counts, in any case.

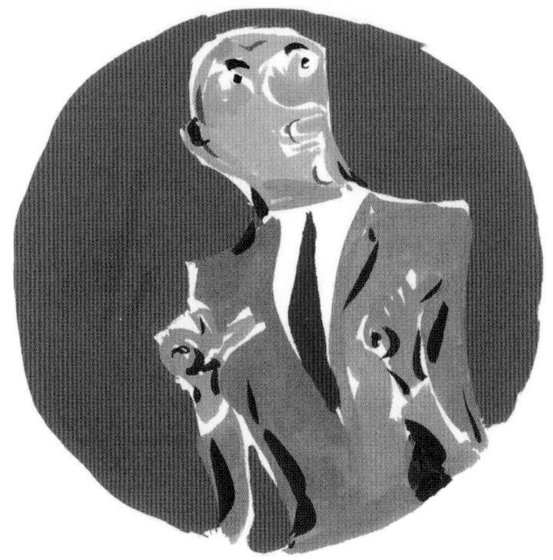

III — 029

THE GRAY SUIT: WHAT FAUX PAS SHOULD YOU AVOID?

Never: 1. Wear it with a steel blue or metallic tie. 2. Wear it with yellow or purple. 3. Wear brown shoes that aren't of equivalent (light/average/dark) intensity. 4. Underestimate the power of green. 5. Underestimate the charm of wine red. 6. Underestimate its effect when combined with a pair of black leather gloves. 7. Miss the chance to wear it with a fine, neutral sweater. 8. Let yourself be convinced that it is old-fashioned when it is just timeless. 9. Forget the aplomb of a cuff. 10. Miss the chance to wear a glen plaid print.

III — 030

Is it ok to layer?

Not only is it ok, layering—which is a science—is what allows us to recognize elegant men. Be careful not to add bulk. Obviously, you'll want to layer your T-shirt, sweater, and cardigan over fresh, clean underwear. Color, whether in an explosion or through a series of matching tones, is a priority. Be careful about choosing prints of different sizes. If you're colorblind, get advice from a trusted friend.

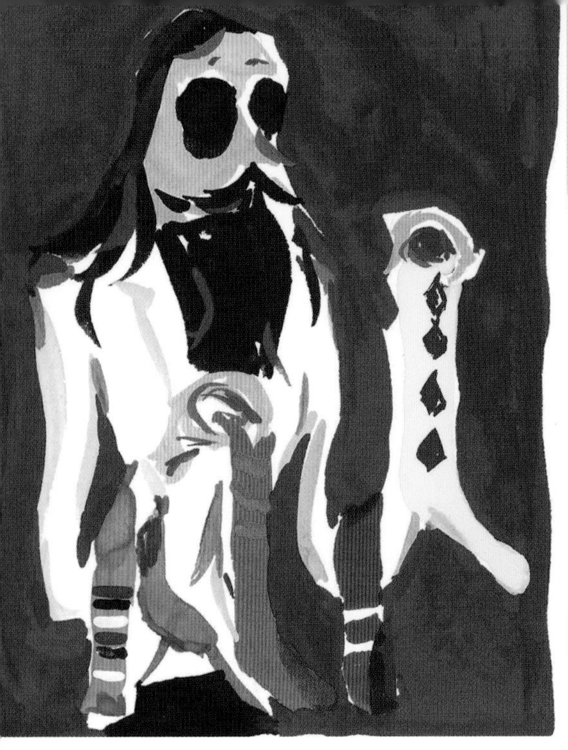

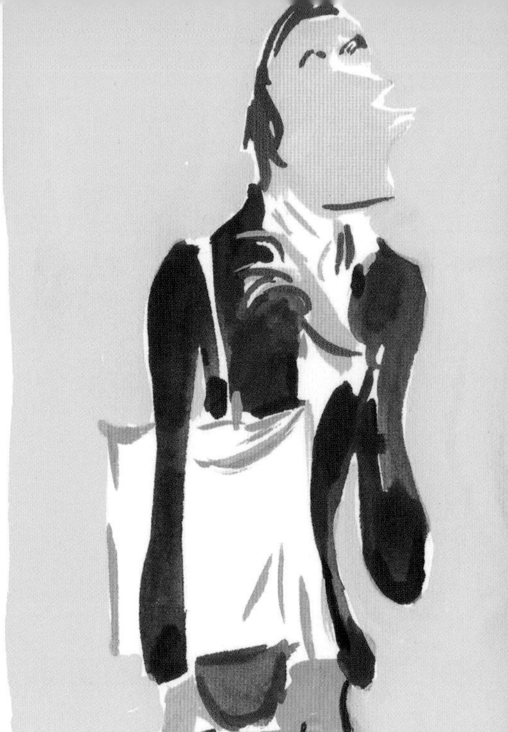

III — 031

HOW CAN YOU CHOOSE THE RIGHT COLOR SOCKS?

Spread the word: a man needs complete freedom when it comes to the color of his socks. Dressing requires enough effort as it is; we should lighten up on the color front. Of course, novelty socks are still out of the question. As for the rest, and even in very formal circumstances, you can do as you please. Otherwise—at the rate we're going—we'll never get there. When in doubt, go for the classic navy blue.

III — 032

Do men still do the carving these days?

This tradition stems, perhaps, from a misguided idea of gallantry. As internationally renowned anthropologist and feminist Françoise Héritier points out, nothing that appears natural to us ever is. With his past roles of hunter and warrior, the dynamic and fervid male remains master of his prey, carving at will.

III — 033

TO TOTE, OR NOT TO TOTE?

A large, unbleached canvas tote bag, whether rectangular or square, can work with different looks. It is advisable not to use one in the city, but keep it for jaunts to the country or beach. Combined with a towel, sunscreen, and a bucket and shovel, the day can at last begin.

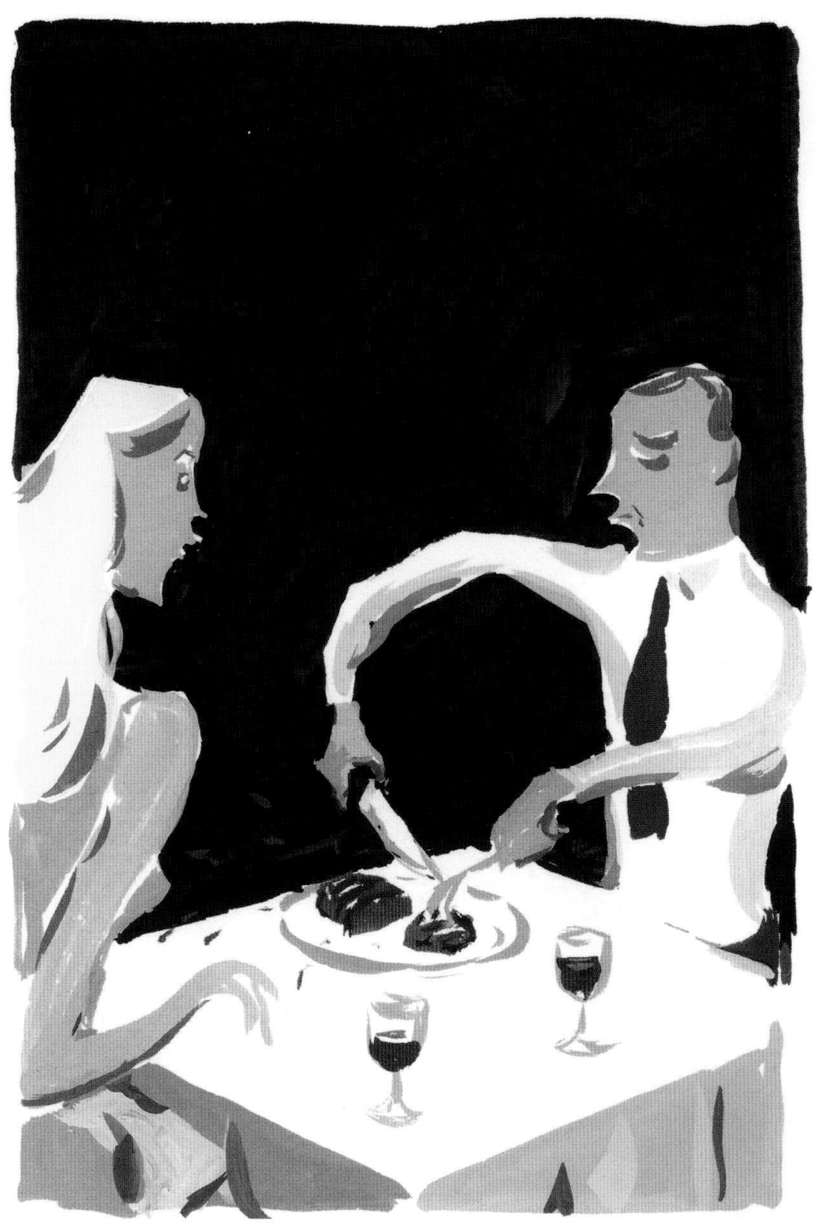

III —— 034

WHITE JEANS OR COLORED CHINOS?

Tread carefully, dear friend, or you might get busted, and we don't like having to play policeman. White jeans are worn with a wide, black leather belt. They are cut straight below the ankle and do not break. Refined types traditionally wear them with loafers (black leather or brown suede) and a blue shirt with rolled-up sleeves. They go very well with any type of jacket except gray—not even very light gray. Colored chinos are younger and look quintessentially American. They're easy to wear with a twist and are worn today in any way whatsoever, with any kind of shoe. They suit any shape, but they must never, for any reason, be worn on a regular basis. Why not? Well, that's a piece of cake: colored chinos provide punctuation.

III —— 035

ARE MILITARY JACKETS A RELIABLE ALLY?

They haven't been since World War II. These days, the military jacket doesn't look cool—it just gives the wearer the vague impression of being hip. Which isn't quite the same thing.

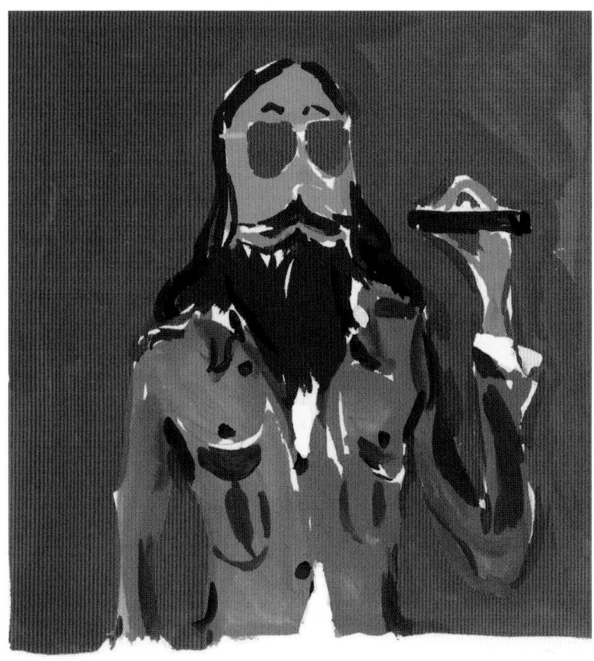

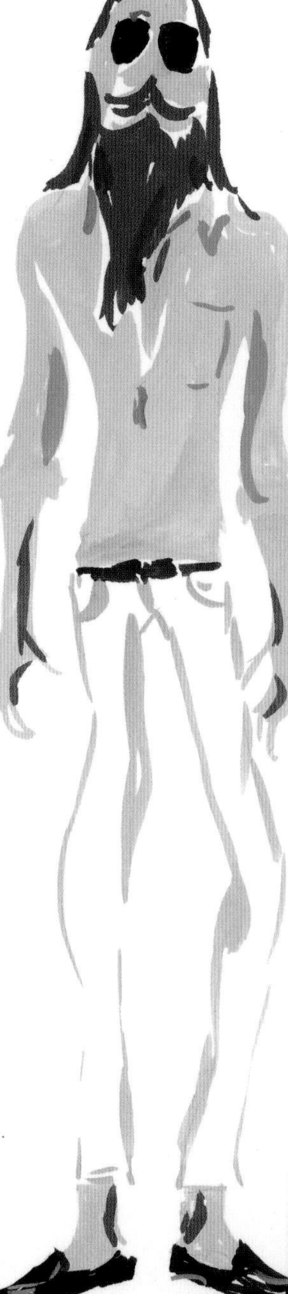

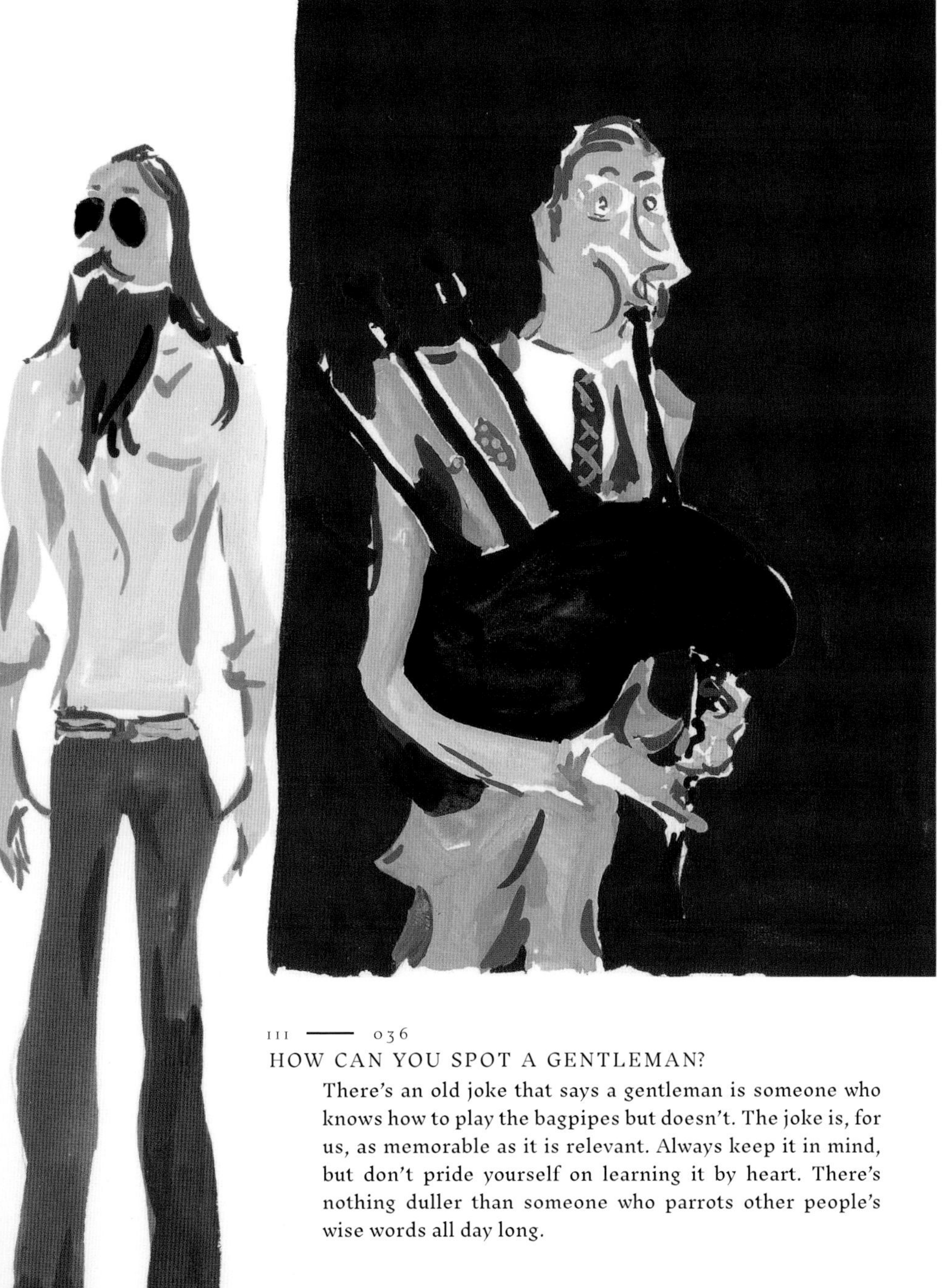

III —— 036

HOW CAN YOU SPOT A GENTLEMAN?

There's an old joke that says a gentleman is someone who knows how to play the bagpipes but doesn't. The joke is, for us, as memorable as it is relevant. Always keep it in mind, but don't pride yourself on learning it by heart. There's nothing duller than someone who parrots other people's wise words all day long.

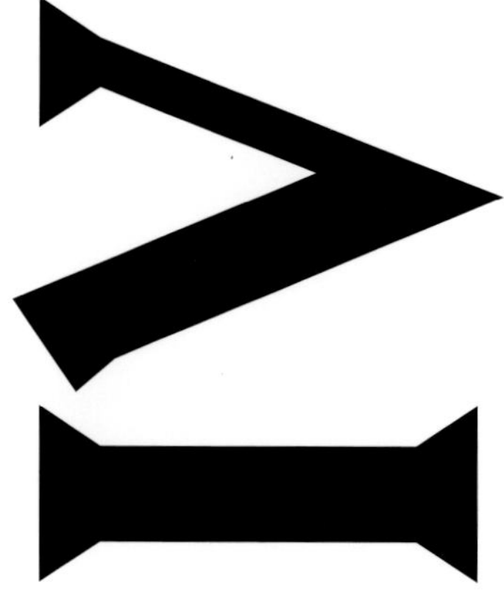

MAKE THE ORDINARY

Are joggers show-offs? • What should every savvy business traveler know? • How can you dress well when you're broke? • How can you make peace with your first gray hair? • What do you wear to smoke a cigar? (Or is smoking cigars just for jerks?) • Would Marcello Mastroianni smoke an electronic cigarette? • What role should you play at a barbecue? • When and how should you cross your legs? • Are faded jeans really back? • How can you conquer stress with style? • What (fashion) ideas should you borrow from women? • Haircuts: scissors or razor? • Can you copy someone

EXTRA-ORDINARY

else's order at a restaurant? • How should you test a cologne? • Should you button up your naval sweater? • Should you wear badges and buttons? • Is it ok to put your hands in your jacket pockets? • What gift should you offer your manager after the summer vacation? • How can you be suave at the supermarket? • What's the coolest place for a tattoo? • Should you lay your beach towel on the sand? • Tempted by a little zentai? • Should you wear patent leather shoes with a tux? • What protocol should you follow at a city bike station?

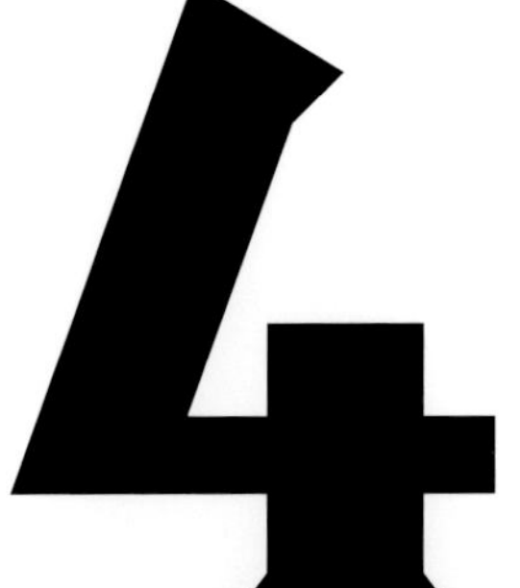

CHAPTER FOUR

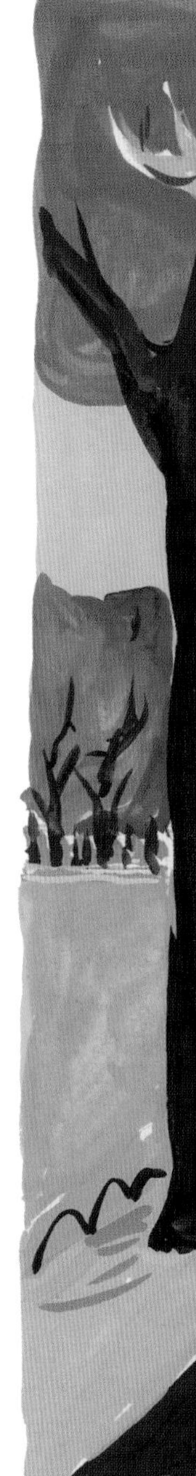

IV — 001

ARE JOGGERS SHOW-OFFS?

In September, during the first week back at work after summer vacation, you promised yourself you'd start exercising again, possibly following the advice of your favorite magazine, *GQ*. A month later, you've lost your motivation. It shows. And on top of that you're depressed. But remember, the city dweller who runs when everyone else is slacking off is valiant and admired—the object of many fantasies. As show-offs never hibernate, it's essential that you grab your Rocky outfit for a public session of squats and lunges.

IV — 002

WHAT SHOULD EVERY SAVVY BUSINESS TRAVELER KNOW?

This author's astute brother—founder of a website dedicated to publishing biographies for the general public (plumedelephant.com)—came up with the following innovation, which, for a very minor investment, will undoubtedly stimulate the business world and finally get global economic growth off the ground again. Hold on to your hat. When a poor devil has to take a red-eye or stay somewhere overnight for work, he packs his pajama T-shirt and an extra pair of boxers in an ordinary expandable file folder with elastic closure. Should the contents of his briefcase spill onto the floor during a meeting (which has never happened before...), he'll be saved from embarrassment. He is thus guaranteed to sign all the contracts in the world, in triplicate, with every page duly initialed. More family secrets are scattered throughout this book.

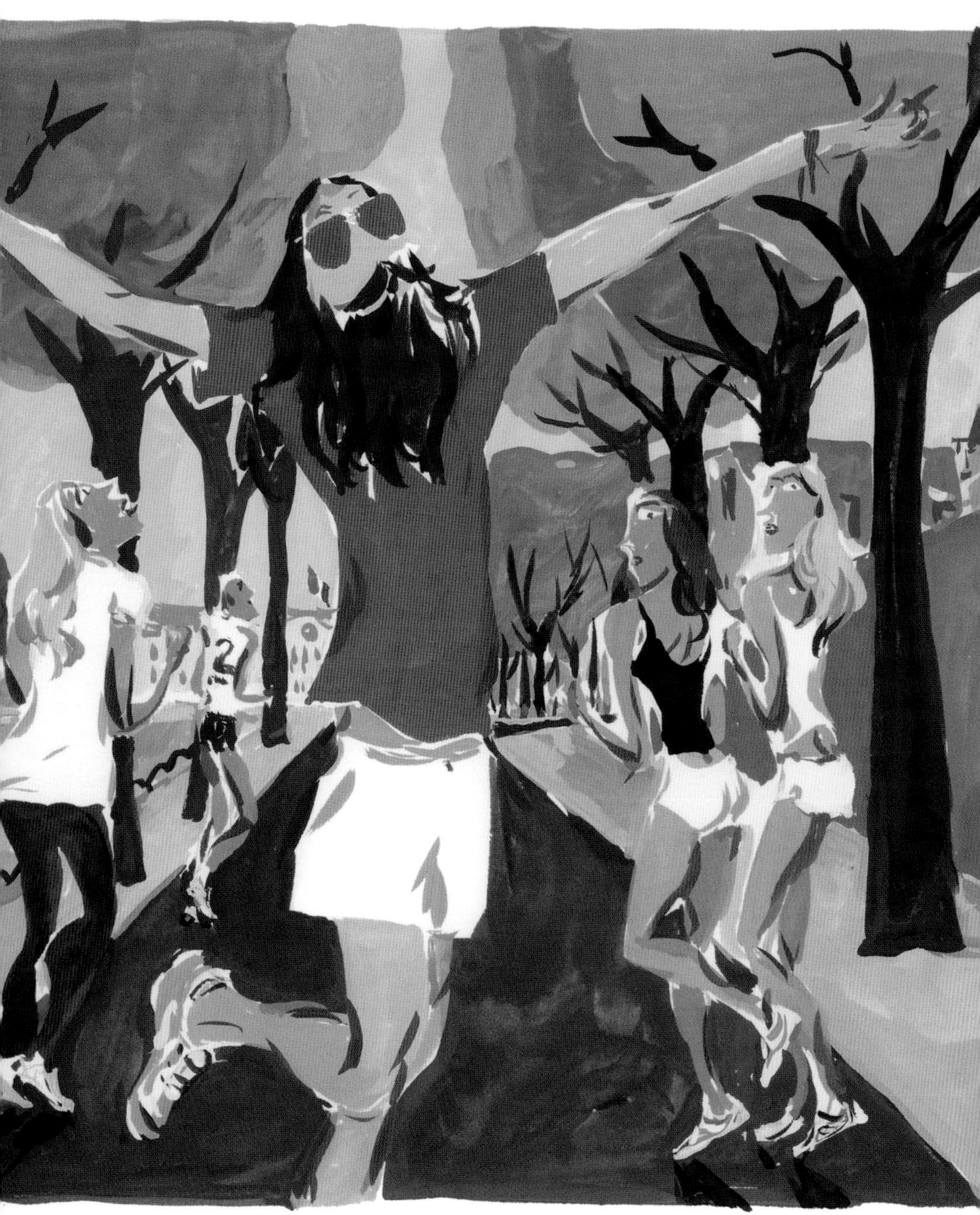

LXXVI

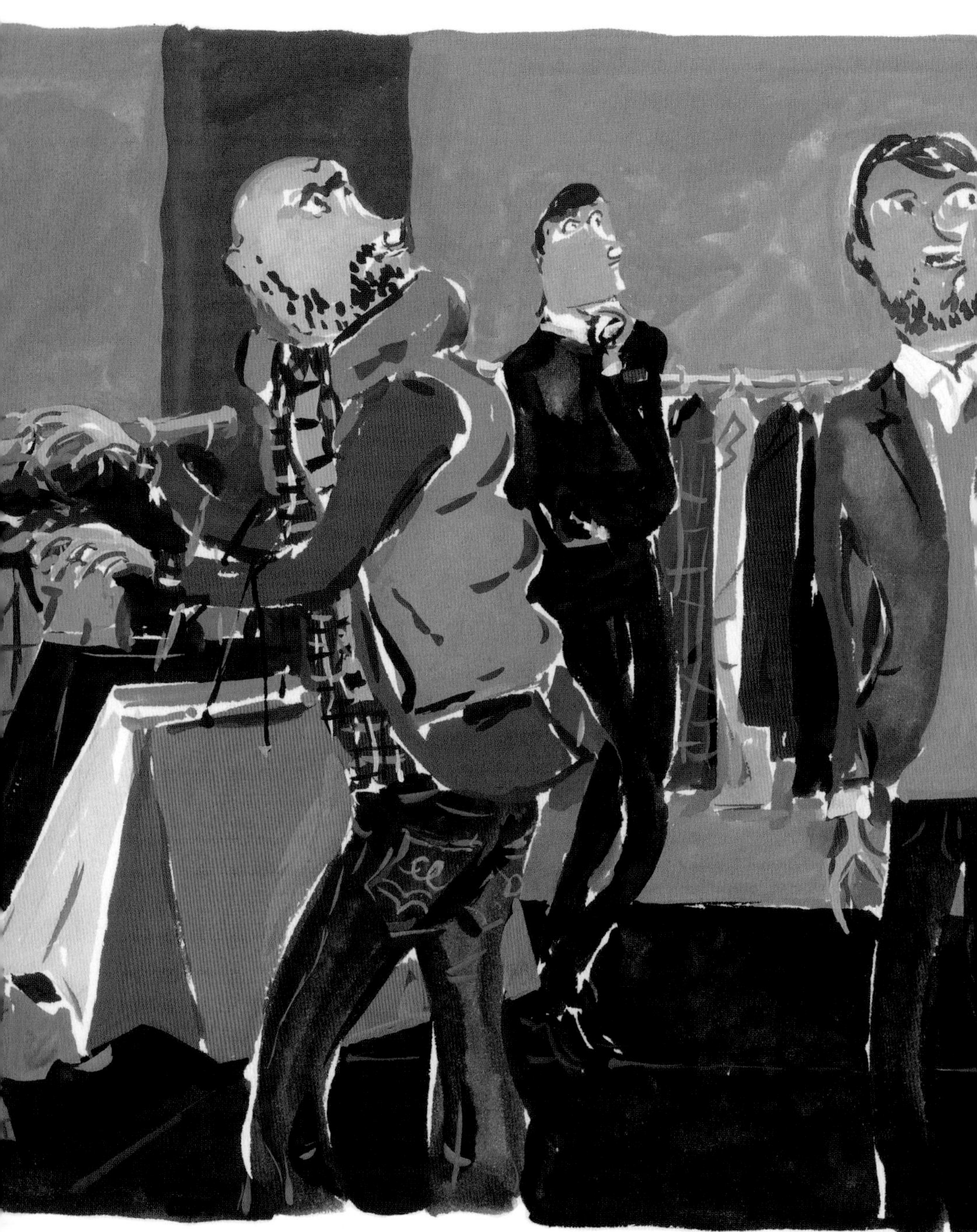

MAKE THE ORDINARY EXTRAORDINARY

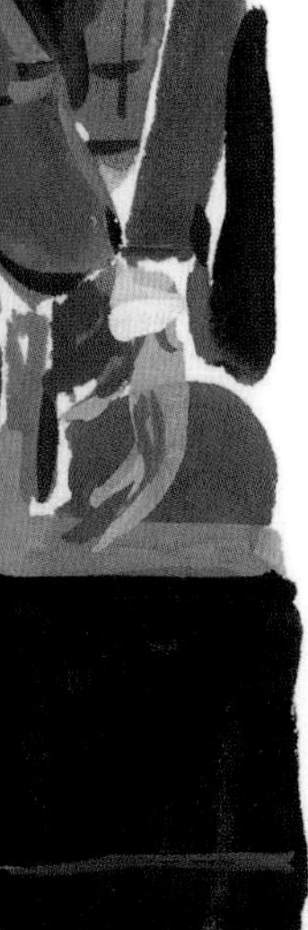

IV — 003

HOW CAN YOU DRESS WELL WHEN YOU'RE BROKE?

You don't have to give up being stylish just because you're on a tight budget. Take a pair of white sneakers, indigo or raw denim jeans (no fancy stitching on the pockets or bad bleach jobs), a few white button-down and polo shirts, a sweater, a fitted jacket—preferably bought on sale from one of the major chains—and you're all set. On a reasonable budget, a man can have a chic, casual, go-anywhere look. Trust us: no one will be able to judge the state of your bank account from this outfit. We can't say the same for your hair. Stay away from overly technical, state-of-the-art, assembly-line cuts that are carried out in cheap hair salons. Yikes, you came within a hair's breadth of that one, didn't you?

IV — 004

How can you make peace with your first gray hair?

There's no point in launching a crusade against this axis of evil; aim instead for neatness. Watching great movie classics should help you identify which silver fox look is just right for you.

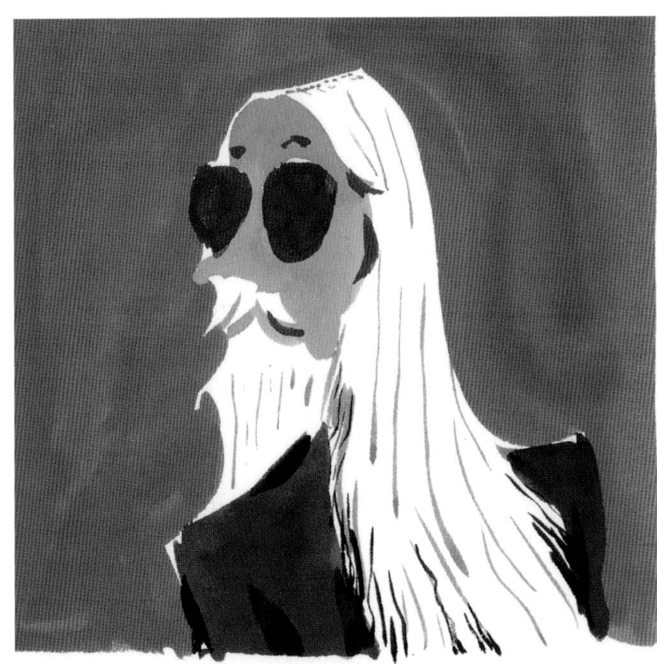

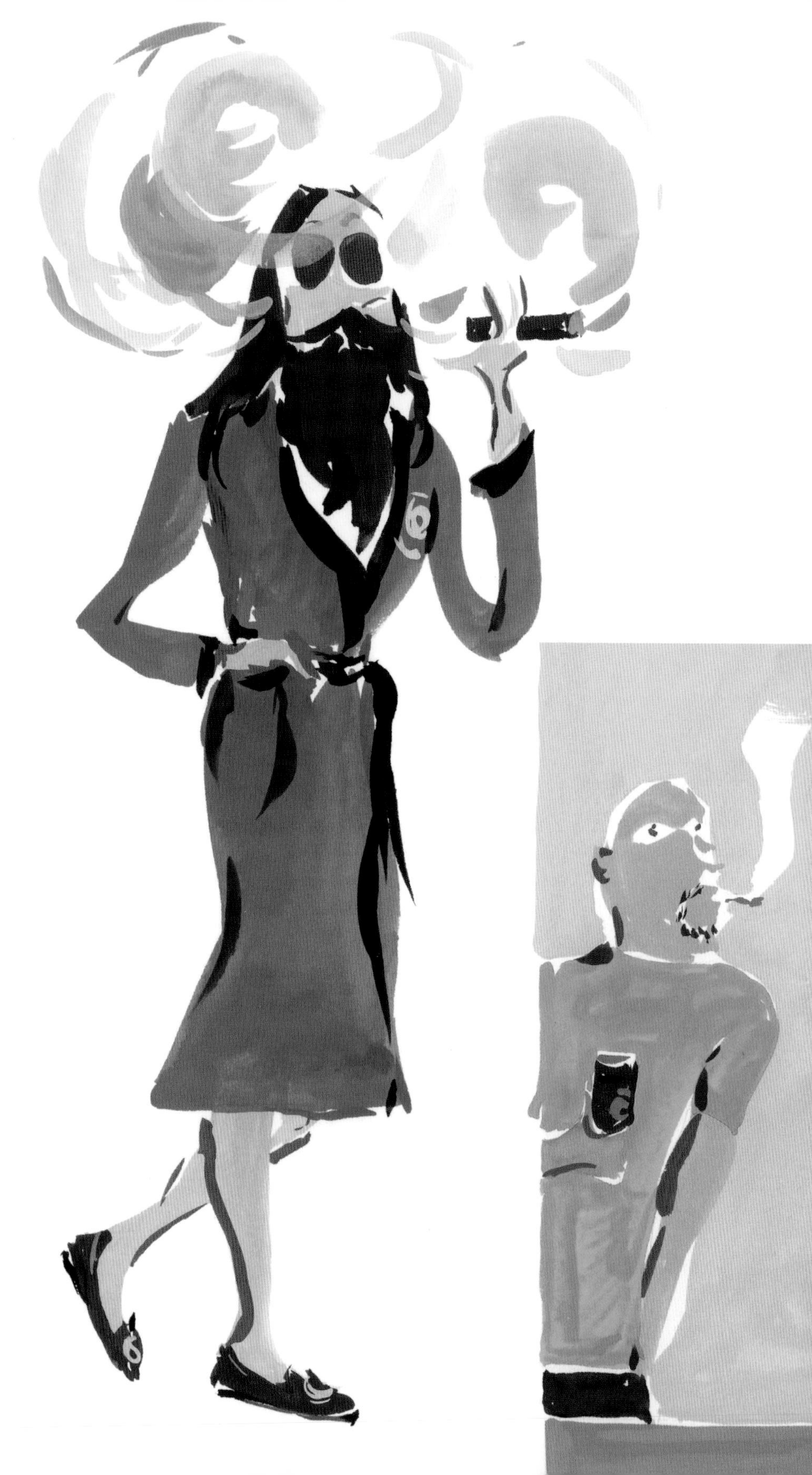

IV —— 005

WHAT DO YOU WEAR TO SMOKE A CIGAR? (OR IS SMOKING CIGARS JUST FOR JERKS?)

Even though 99 percent of cigar smokers are considered huge jackasses, if not mentally challenged, we are taking into account here the fringe population that sees cigar-smoking as a type of meditation, with the power to pull you out of your daily routine. We have even smoked a few cigars ourselves, on various occasions, believe it or not. As for your outfit, you'll wear silk pajamas, robe, and slippers; a striped, double-breasted suit; or a tux. Being over fifty is (always) a plus. Never have your photo taken with a cigar in your mouth. Always smoke calmly, with one hand in your pocket.

IV —— 006

Would Marcello Mastroianni smoke an electronic cigarette?

When a style question gnaws at you, all you have to do is ask yourself what Marcello Mastroianni would do. Clunky and hard to hold, e-cigarettes are impossible to smoke elegantly. Mastroianni, vaping, just wouldn't have had the same seductive edge (or the same serious look behind the steering wheel). In short, e-smokes are a tad cartoonish, *à la* Tex Avery, so you'll have to adjust the way you vape. If necessary, invest in a long black model with a cap, so you'll look less like you're sucking on a pen.

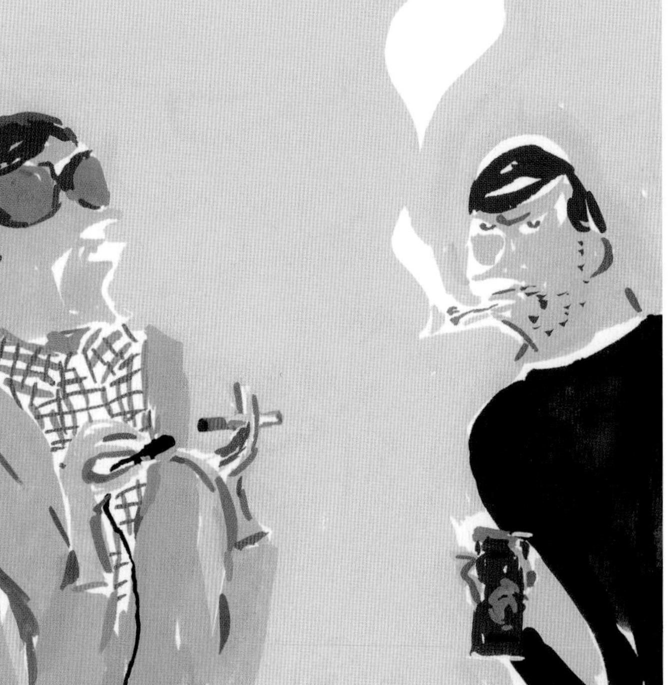

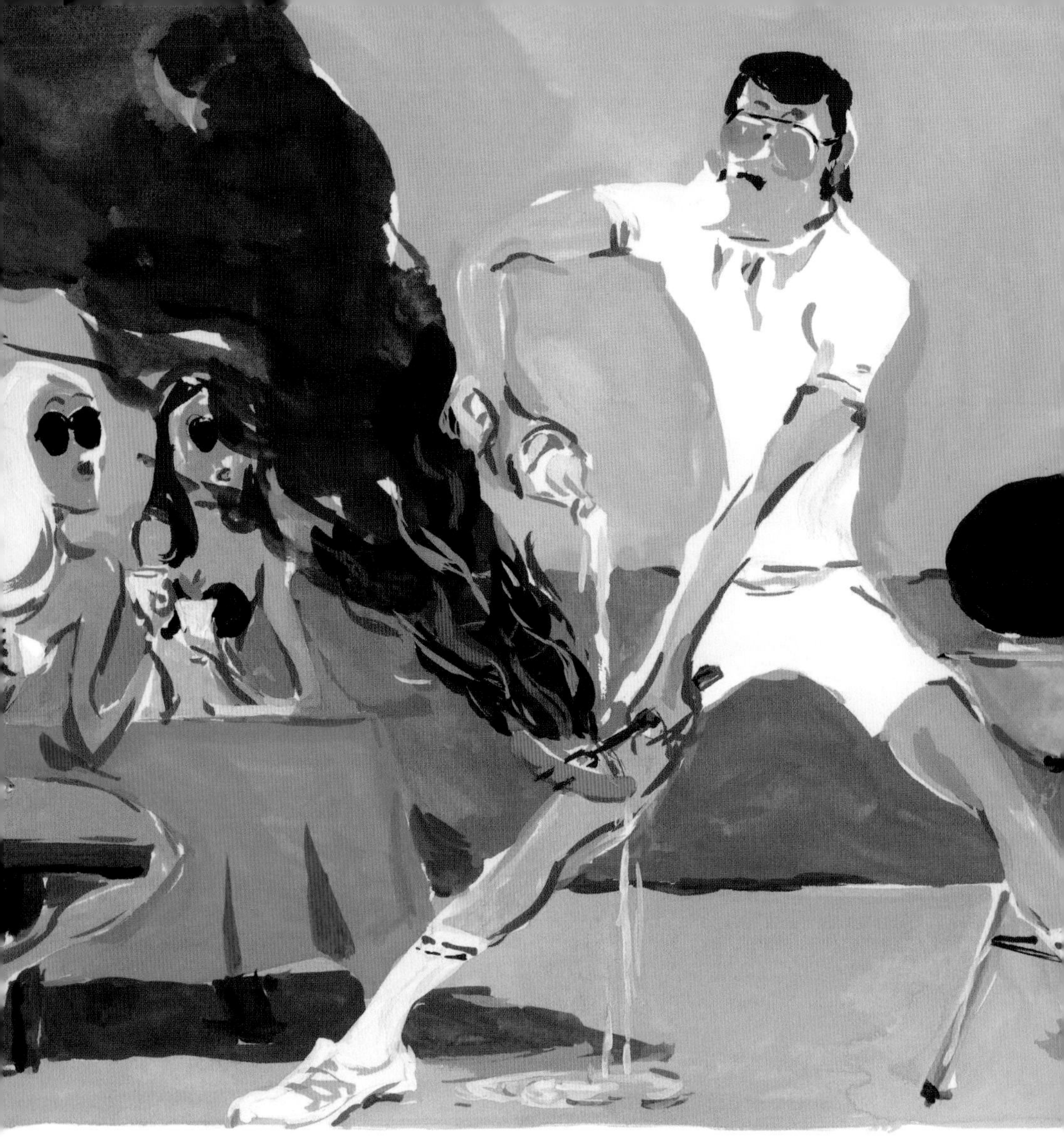

IV —— 007

WHAT ROLE SHOULD YOU PLAY AT A BARBECUE?

At this kind of gathering, you should take a key role at the start by firing up the grill, and at the end by serving the barbecued meats. Saddling yourself with the cooking is of no interest whatsoever, unless you want the fumes to slowly asphyxiate you. If you're stuck coughing, with a headlamp strapped to your forehead to help you distinguish between the charred sausages and the ones that have burnt to a cinder, you've had it—especially since, once everyone is seated, no one ever really thanks the cook. They're all too busy devouring what's left to eat. Finally, don't be that guy who pretends to be busy when he hasn't actually been given any responsibility. You deserve better. So pour everyone a glass of rosé.

IV —— 008

WHEN AND HOW SHOULD YOU CROSS YOUR LEGS?

You're really getting down to the nitty-gritty today. Yes, like it or not, it has been declared that sitting with your legs crossed is the *only* way to sit this summer. Why? There's no harm in asking. For the simple reason that it allows you to hang around on an outdoor table at your local watering hole without looking like a loser. Face it, it really isn't very elegant to keep both feet on the ground when you're seated, except when the table has a higher function (meal, bridge, quiet aperitif). So you have no choice but to cross your legs the rest of the time. It's an inflexible rule, easy to remember, and applies only if the following advice is respected. There are two distinct styles for crossing your legs: the *GQ* style, and the other style. 1. The *GQ* style: the knees overlap perfectly. The foot hangs free (it is not tucked behind the calf in an ungainly fashion) and retains its panache. Placed judiciously, so as not to bother anyone, it arcs itself gently to free up the passageway at any moment. This position is, of course, suitable for all circumstances. 2. The other style: one leg rests suspended on the knee of the other leg. This creates a 45° angle, which is intolerable (the maximum tolerated is 20°). It may be fun, but it is not a posture for those who are building a better world.

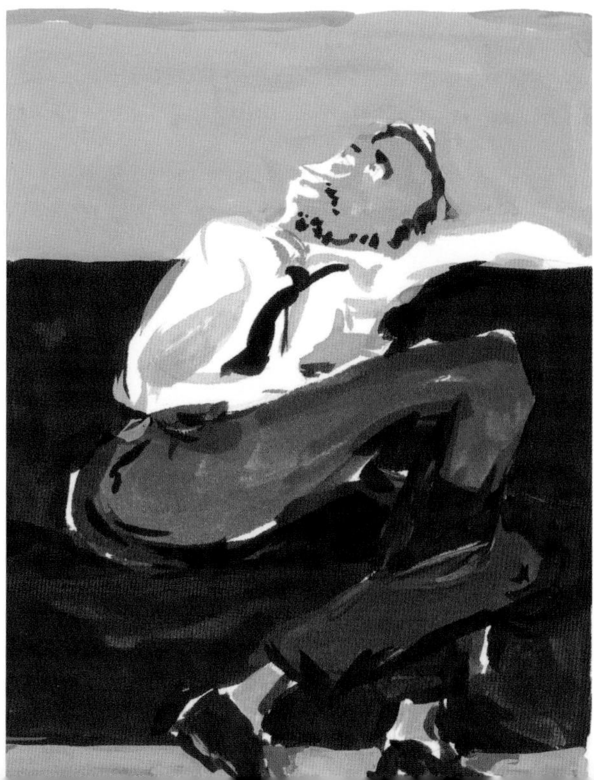

IV —— 009

ARE FADED JEANS REALLY BACK?

Yes—even if the bleached look that came back didn't last that long. By "bleached," we mean garments that have that wasted look. Let's say you were cleaning the kitchen and spilled cleaning products all over yourself, and blobs of paint fell on you, too. The coolest guy in the world would say to himself, "Great, I'll look even grungier than ever." The *GQ* man says, "I'm going to pass these jeans on to my girlfriend; she'll know how to make them work, and I have that damn PowerPoint presentation to finish." However, rest assured that faded jeans are popular again. By adopting raw denim jeans as the uniform of the service industry, turning them into the new ordinary, we've made the faded, "pre-worn," ripped style even more desirable. Every summer, they gain more ground; now available in all the stores, they are accessible to the faceless masses. Wearing worn-out jeans today is a way of proudly making a statement.

IV —— 010

How can you conquer stress with style?

A pocket square in your jacket leads the eye toward your chest, meaning no one's looking at your stomach. A pocket square is also useful when you want to wipe your hands prior to a decisive handshake. On the night before a peak stress-causing event, get your outfit ready ahead of time. Don't be late because you have to iron it.

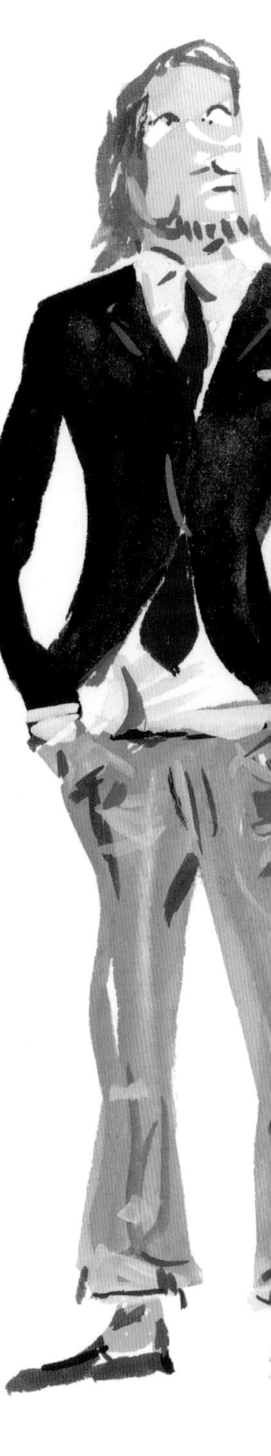

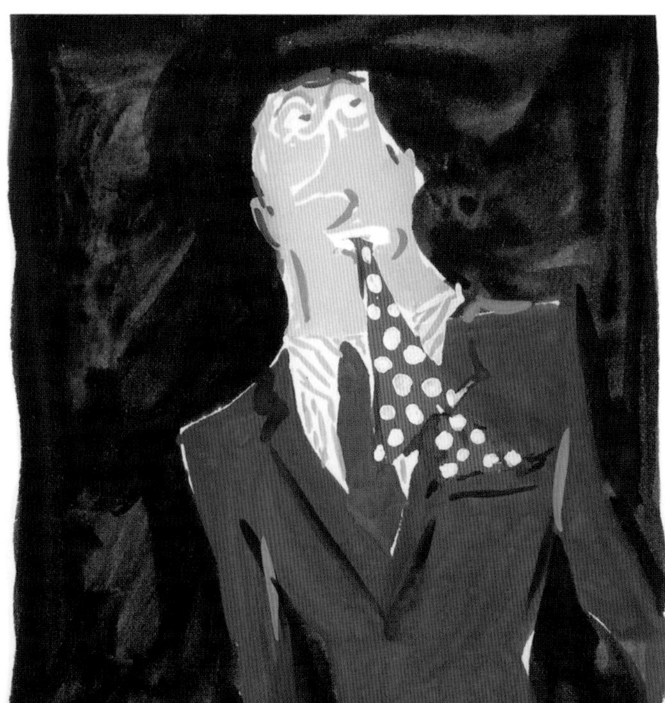

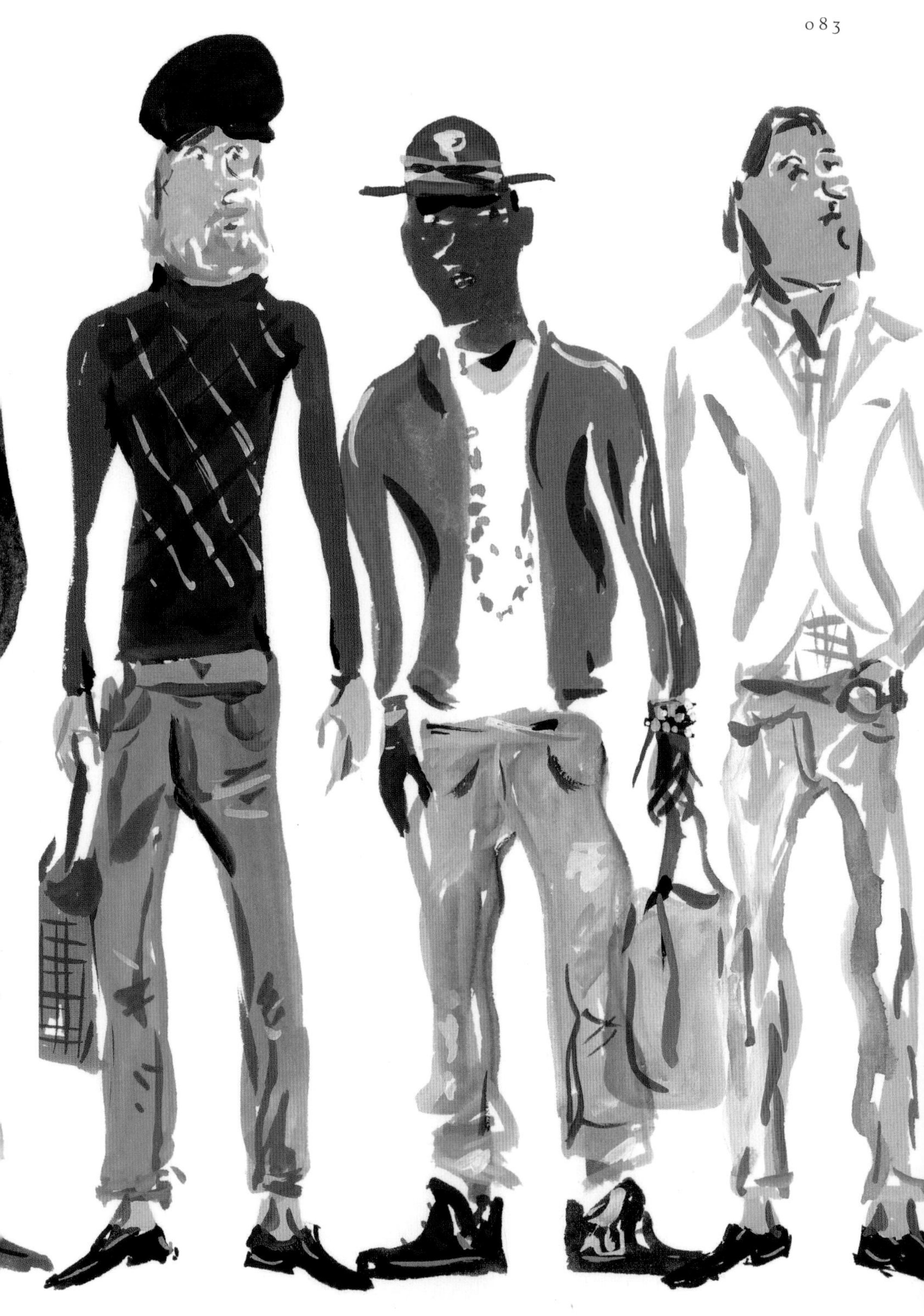

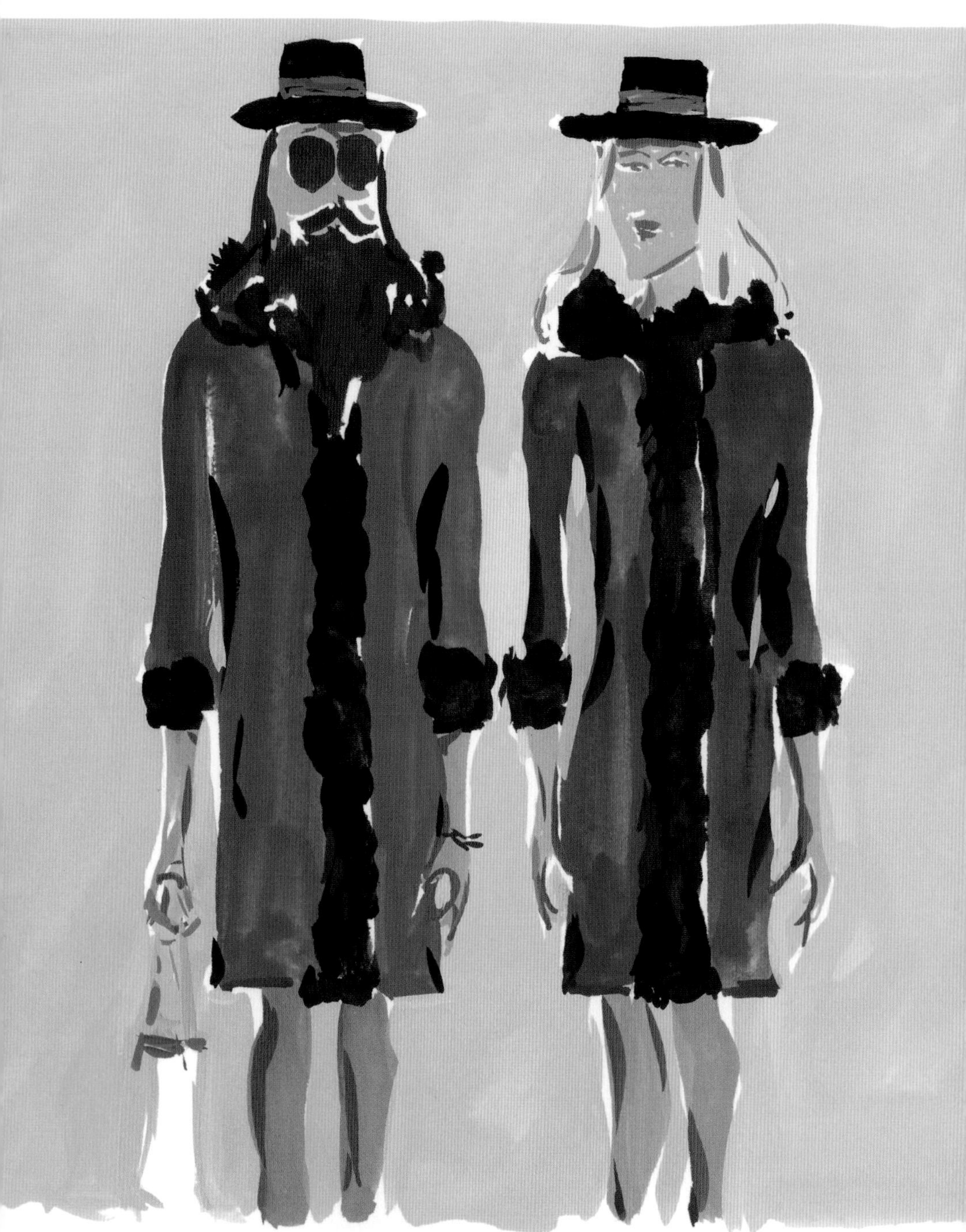

MAKE THE ORDINARY EXTRAORDINARY

IV — 011

WHAT (FASHION) IDEAS SHOULD YOU BORROW FROM WOMEN?

Dear friends, women's trends are more or less the same as ours: the 1960s for a Pop or Beat look; the 1970s for a sensual, hippy vibe; a military look for braving the cold as an *Übermensch*; and the 1980s–90s for subtly slumming it. Anything goes. Anything at all.

IV — 012

HAIRCUTS: SCISSORS OR RAZOR?

No question: scissors will help you steer clear of standardized trendy cuts. If a barber uses scissors only, you're guaranteed to spend an hour in a comfy barber's chair, with no itchy little hairs left on your neck when you leave. Most of all, you can be sure you'll have an immaculate haircut that will draw nothing but compliments.

IV — 013

CAN YOU COPY SOMEONE ELSE'S ORDER AT A RESTAURANT?

You're so undecided that, when the time comes to order, you end up going for the same choice as your person of reference (generally your boss): a rare sirloin steak. Depending on the context, this simple act of currying favor could earn you a few biting remarks at the coffee machine, confirming your reputation as a premium a*@-kisser. Just order the simplest thing on the menu next time.

IV — 014

How should you test a cologne?

In the store, spray your aroma of choice onto a strip of card. Apply the lucky winner to your skin, then walk around the block twice. Sniff again. Reenter the shop and make a decision!

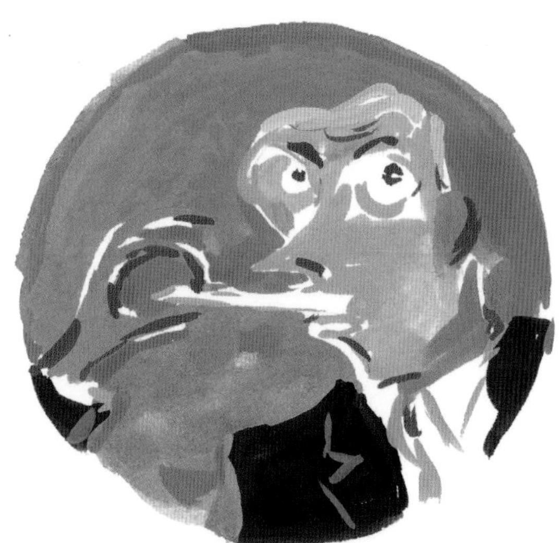

IV —— 015

Should you button up your naval sweater?

The question of buttoning doesn't seem all that fundamental to us, so we accept two opposing scenarios:

1. Totally unbuttoned to offset the tubular look of this garment, which tightly hugs the torso the way a sock does the calf.

2. Totally buttoned up to accentuate the space-suit effect and add firmness to a part of the body that sometimes lacks it.

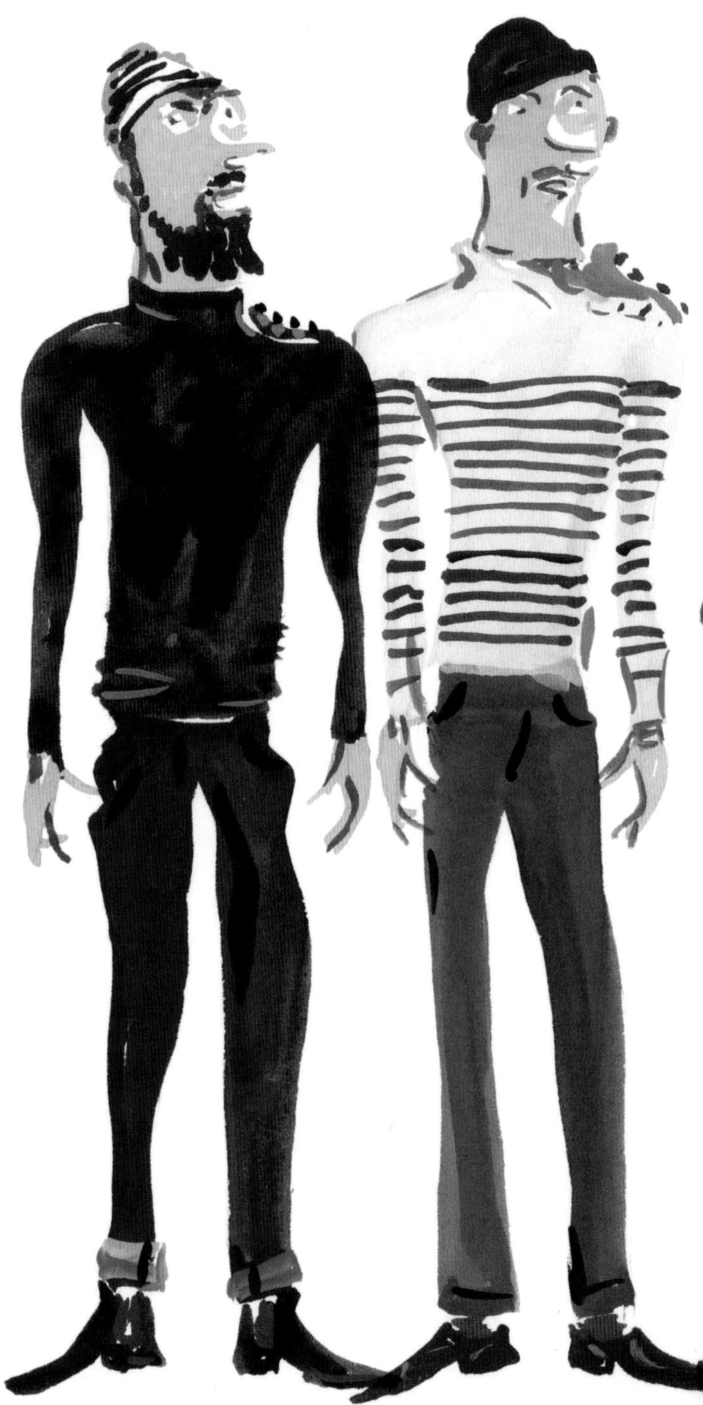

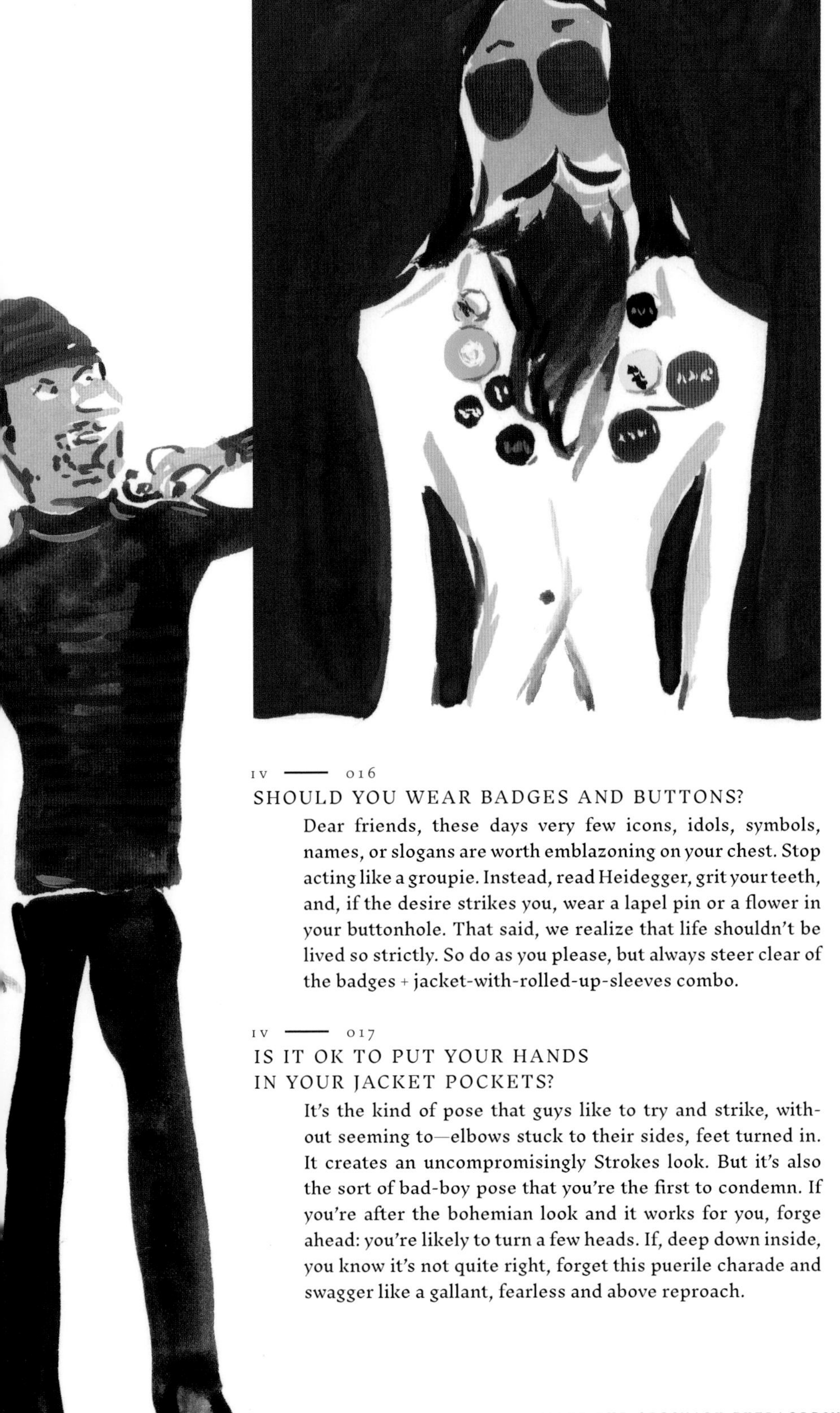

IV —— 016

SHOULD YOU WEAR BADGES AND BUTTONS?

Dear friends, these days very few icons, idols, symbols, names, or slogans are worth emblazoning on your chest. Stop acting like a groupie. Instead, read Heidegger, grit your teeth, and, if the desire strikes you, wear a lapel pin or a flower in your buttonhole. That said, we realize that life shouldn't be lived so strictly. So do as you please, but always steer clear of the badges + jacket-with-rolled-up-sleeves combo.

IV —— 017

IS IT OK TO PUT YOUR HANDS IN YOUR JACKET POCKETS?

It's the kind of pose that guys like to try and strike, without seeming to—elbows stuck to their sides, feet turned in. It creates an uncompromisingly Strokes look. But it's also the sort of bad-boy pose that you're the first to condemn. If you're after the bohemian look and it works for you, forge ahead: you're likely to turn a few heads. If, deep down inside, you know it's not quite right, forget this puerile charade and swagger like a gallant, fearless and above reproach.

IV —— 018

WHAT GIFT SHOULD YOU OFFER YOUR MANAGER AFTER THE SUMMER VACATION?

A nice little golf kit for the office is always appreciated and doesn't cost much. It enables your boss to work on his putt, to better manage his stress, and, hey, to do something productive during the day. Which is no small thing.

IV —— 019

HOW CAN YOU BE SUAVE AT THE SUPERMARKET?

Grocery shopping is torture. The people depress you, but nevertheless, keep on the straight and narrow. Don't leave your shopping cart in the middle of the aisle. At the cash register, elderly—and smiling—people, beautiful women, and customers with far fewer items than you have priority. Say hello to the checkout person. Keep your means of payment handy. Take the receipt that is handed to you, even if you're not the type to scrutinize it later. Then say goodbye to the checkout person after you've told them an amusing anecdote.

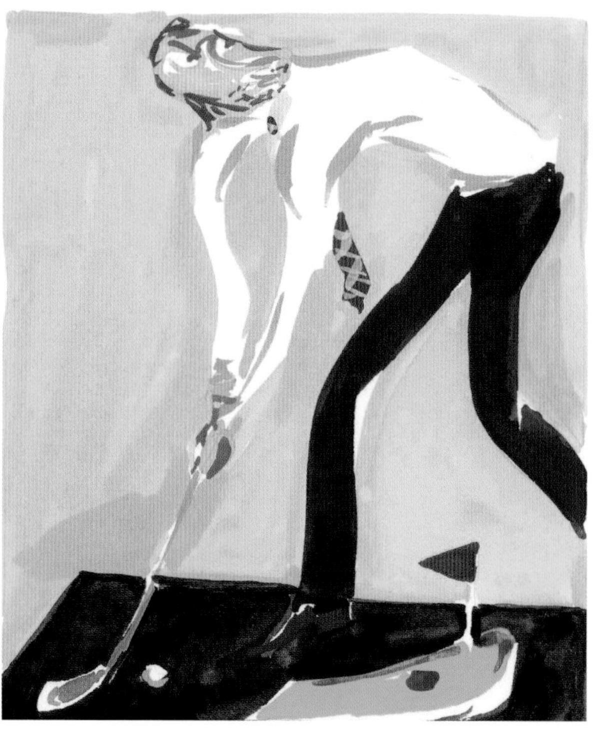

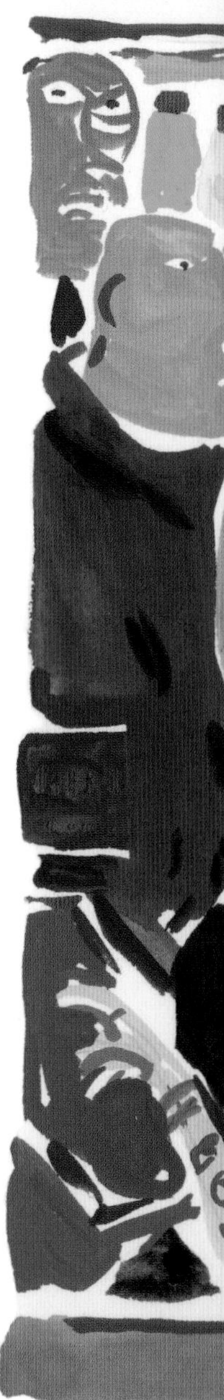

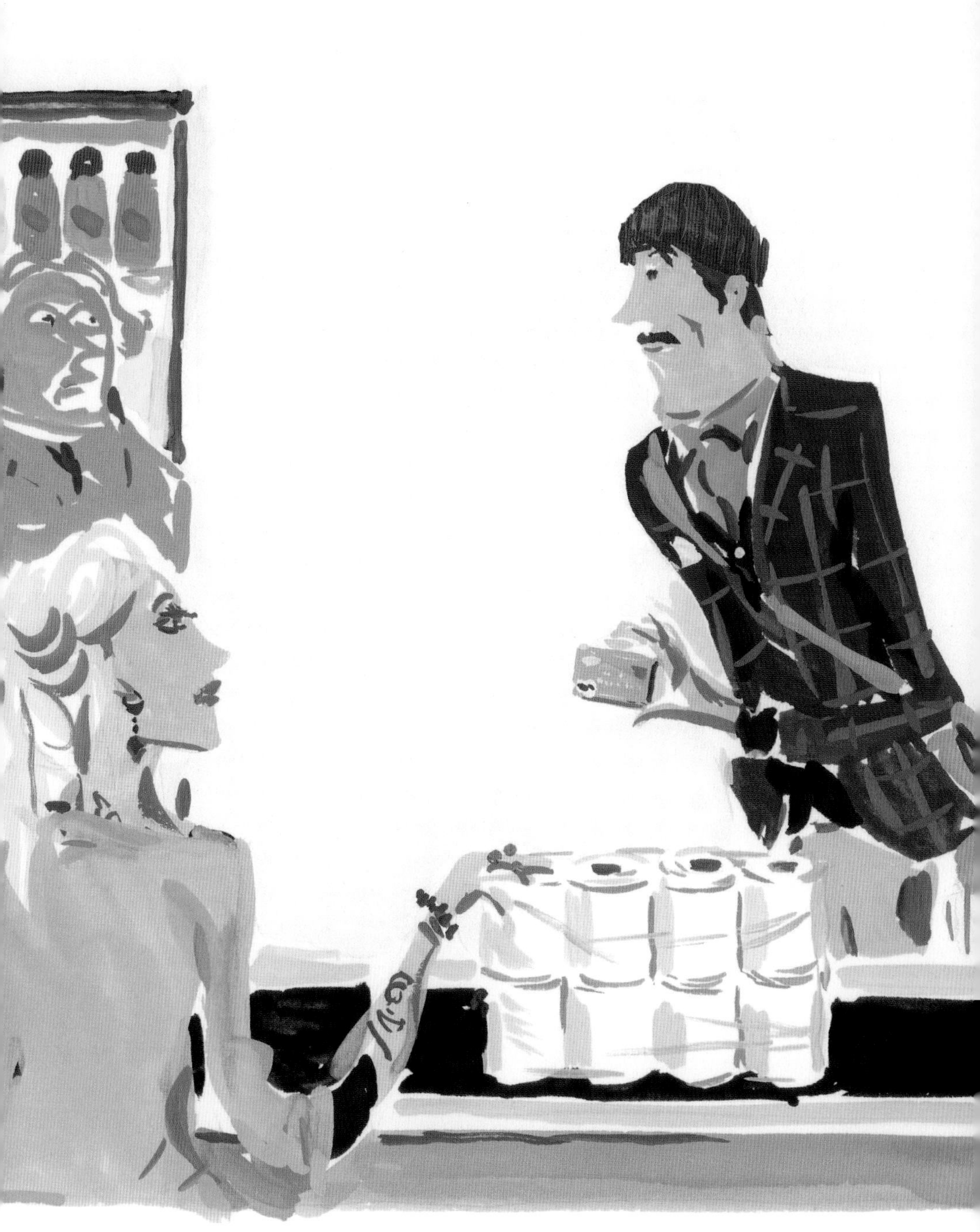

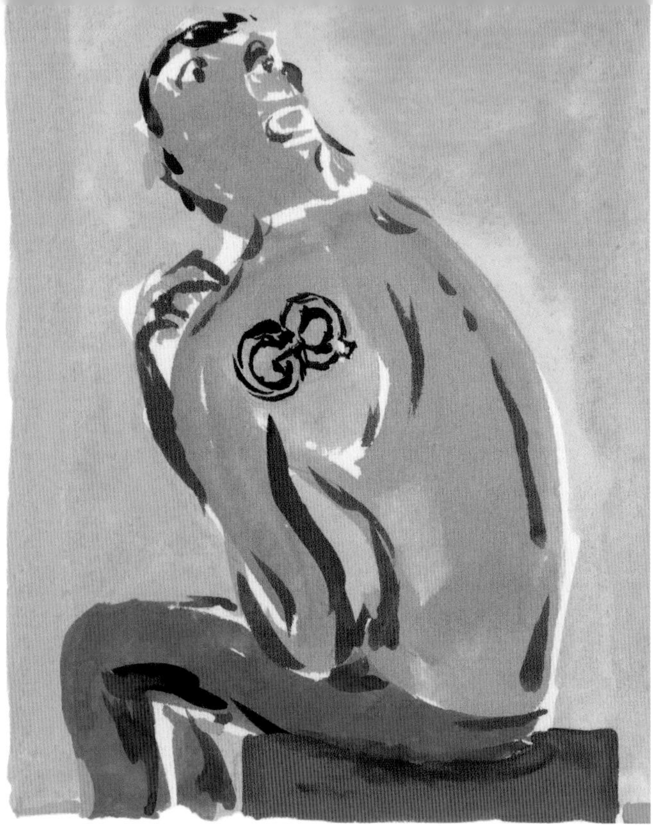

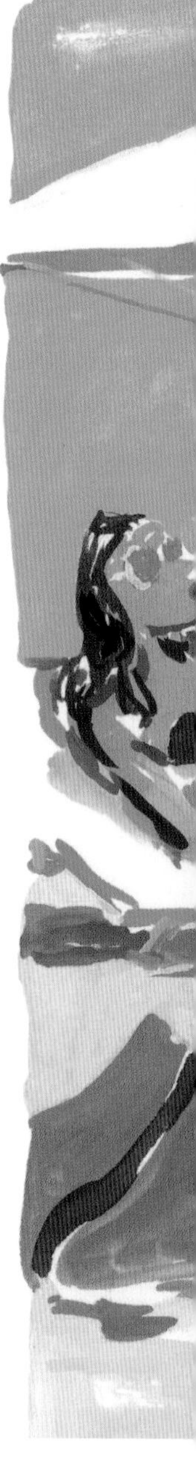

IV —— 020

WHAT'S THE COOLEST PLACE FOR A TATTOO?

Because some of you will take the leap in spite of our reticence, let's try and limit the damage. Our first reflex would have been to go straight for a design on the chest. But the risk is that you'd soon tire of seeing it (backwards) in the bathroom mirror every time you step out of the shower. And on the sternum, guys, it's going to hurt big-time. On the calf, the unavoidable risk is evoking a "Phuket Full Moon Party" atmosphere, circa 1993. Rather than the forearm or biceps, we recommend the shoulder or shoulder blade—it's an area that is particularly easy to show, hide, and forget. To our knowledge, apart from the face—extremely hardcore—there is no special significance to getting a tattoo in one place or another. The fact remains that, wherever it is, a tribal tattoo will inevitably make you look like an adult-film star.

IV —— 021

Should you lay your beach towel on the sand?

Beaches covered with lounge chairs and imbeciles lying around irritate us. It is preferable to take a towel and place it on the sand at a reasonable distance from your neighbors. May they ever gaze upon you, the perfect gentleman.

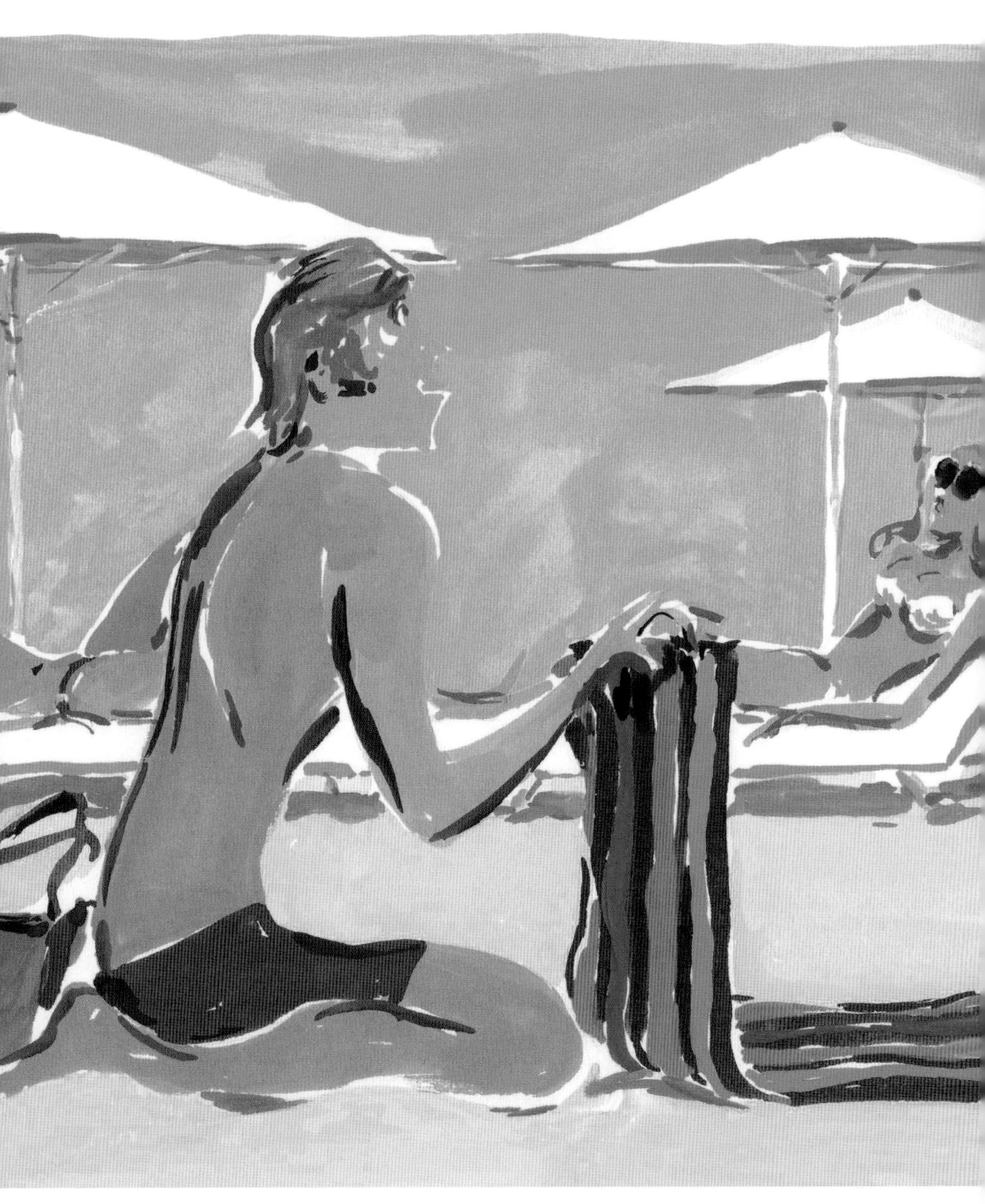

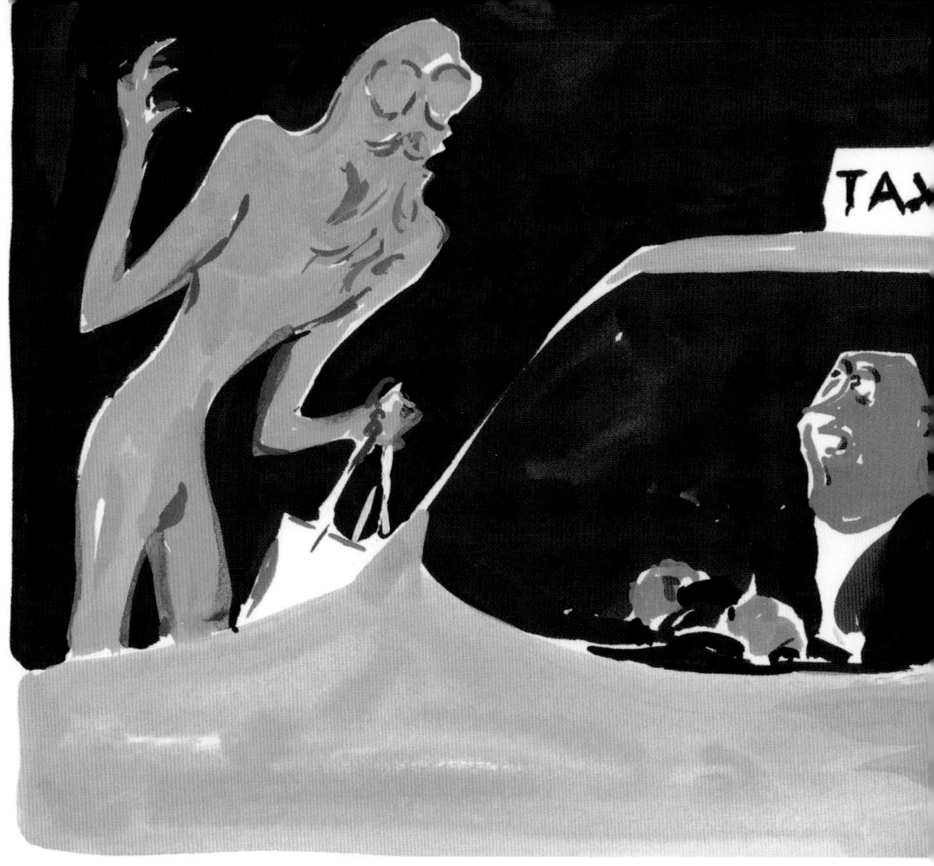

IV —— 022

TEMPTED BY A LITTLE *ZENTAI*?

Should you go for it? Yes, and without any hesitation. If a better disguise exists, we don't know what it is. Well, in fact we do—when someone showed up with a bandaged nose one evening. It looked great with a pair of Martian antennae. Anyway: the *zentai*. This elasthane (rather than latex) jumpsuit covering the entire body has been the subject of special fascination in Japan for twenty years or so. Here, far from S&M circles, the outfit is worn mostly by soccer fans. Whatever the case, when you're wearing your jumpsuit you'll be free to act as a monochrome gentleman. But remember, although people won't necessarily know who you are, it doesn't mean you get to do any old thing you want. And, in the name of all that is decent, wear briefs. Ok, now you can go play.

IV —— 023

Should you wear patent leather shoes with a tux?

A young man at the last Cannes Film Festival (were you there too?) asked our advice on this point. The professional renting him the suit didn't encourage it, which was rather irresponsible on his part.

IV —— 024

WHAT PROTOCOL SHOULD YOU FOLLOW AT A CITY BIKE STATION?

Three categories of renters have emerged. No matter which city you're in, the worst are those who never line their bike up properly and try to force the plug into the available stand. A slightly less egregious group consists of guys who pull away without waiting for the signal that indicates everything is in good order. The third group comprises those who wait patiently until this step has been completed. These are the people who get our support. But to stay looking cool at all times, don't stand around with your head down and hands on your hips. Please, anything but that!

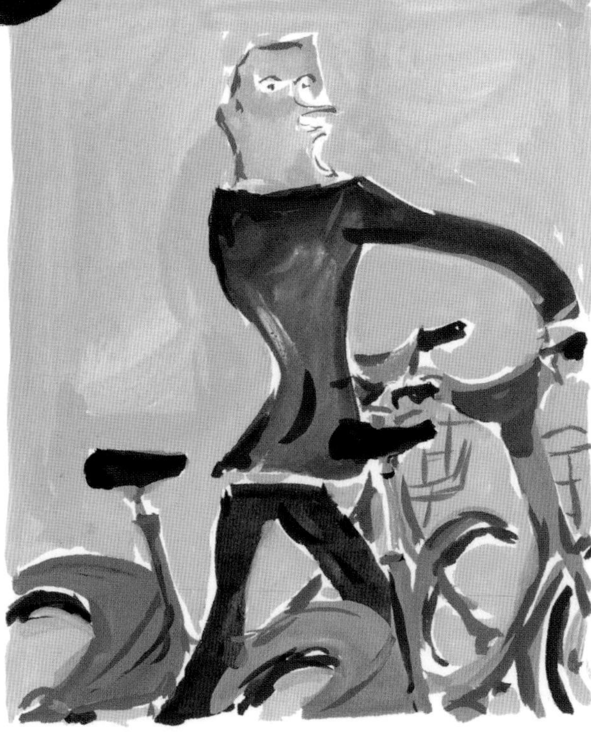

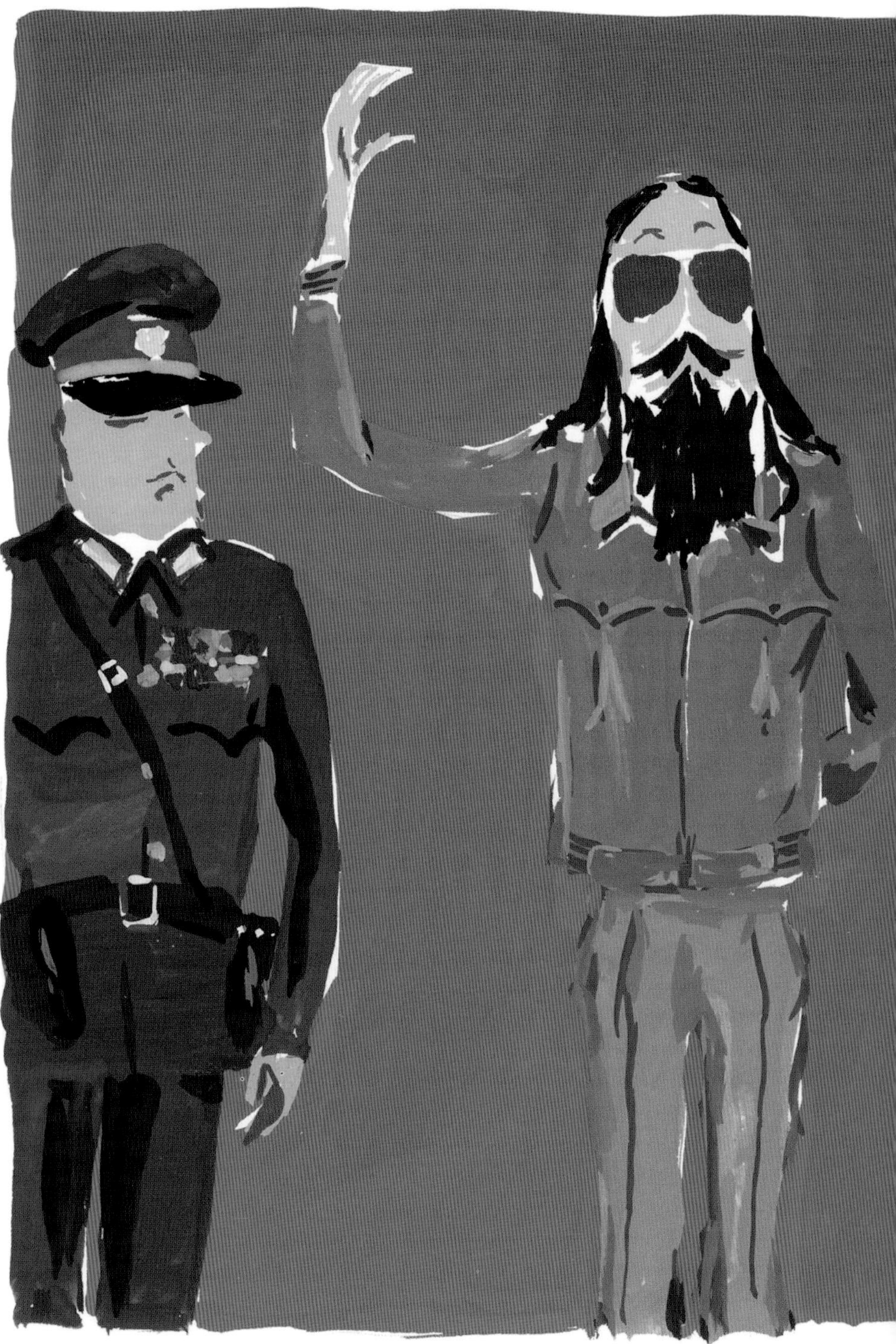

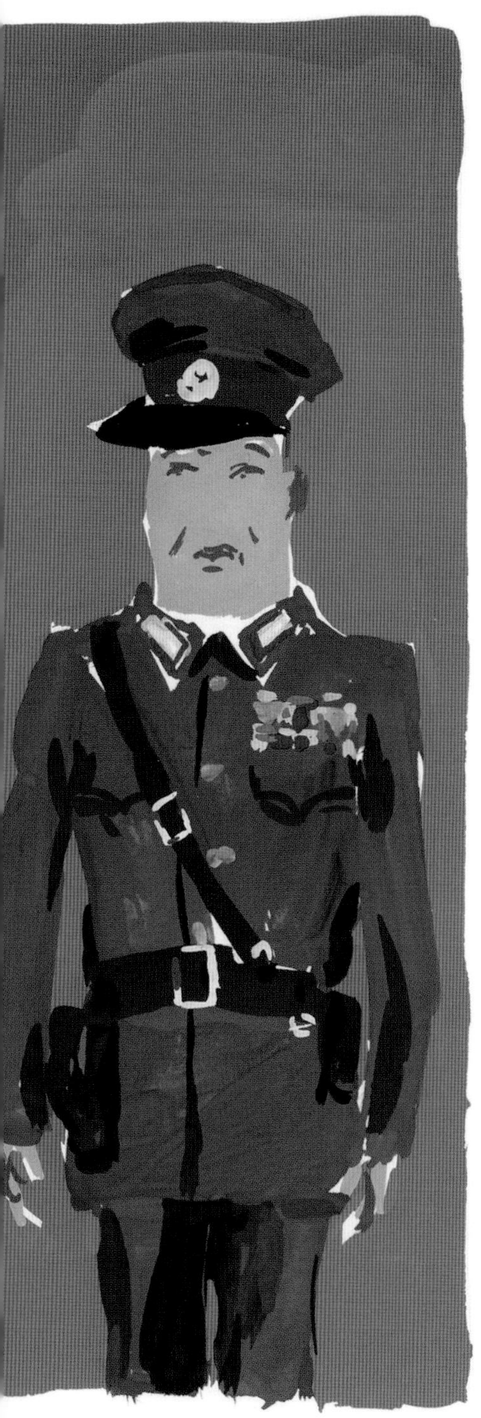

INTERLUDE

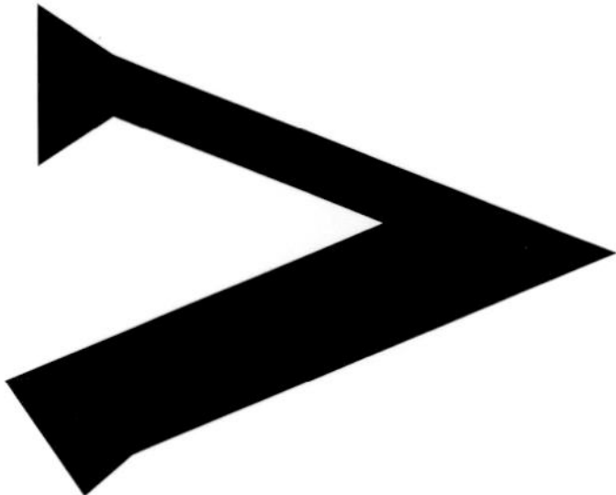

THROW CAUTION TO

V —— 001 › V —— 027

When can you wear a calypso shirt? • Can you wear the T-shirt if you never ever listen to the band? • Should men wear medals? • How can you avoid getting lost in the sartorial woods this winter? • Do real men ride kick scooters? • How can you tell if you've arrived late for a dinner? • Where should you hide your handkerchief when you have a runny nose? • What pet should you get? • How should you dress for a Halloween party? • Is it time for a pocket square comeback? • What's the new kilt? • Why on earth would you hang up your neckties? • Should you tuck in your sweater? • How should you dress for a trip overseas? • Should you take off your glasses when you kiss somebody

THE WIND

on the cheek? • Will a camel-colored coat make it through the winter tundra? • Should we stop wearing fur-trimmed hoods? • Why do some European luxury hotels ring a bell at six o'clock in the morning? • How can you look suave when taking a toke? • Is it ok to splash around with a mask and snorkel? • Can you wear shorts to a beachside restaurant? • Which sport will be on trend this summer? • How can you keep a train car to yourself? • What's the best way to dry an umbrella? • What's the one piece of clothing that every perfect gentleman needs? • How can you look like a boss in Grand Theft Auto V? • What's the best way to wear overalls?

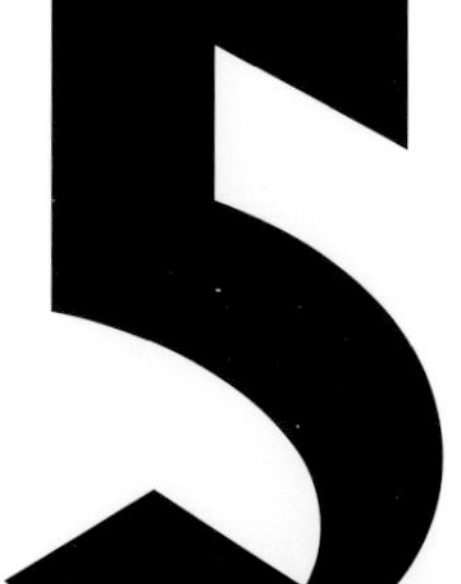

CHAPTER FIVE

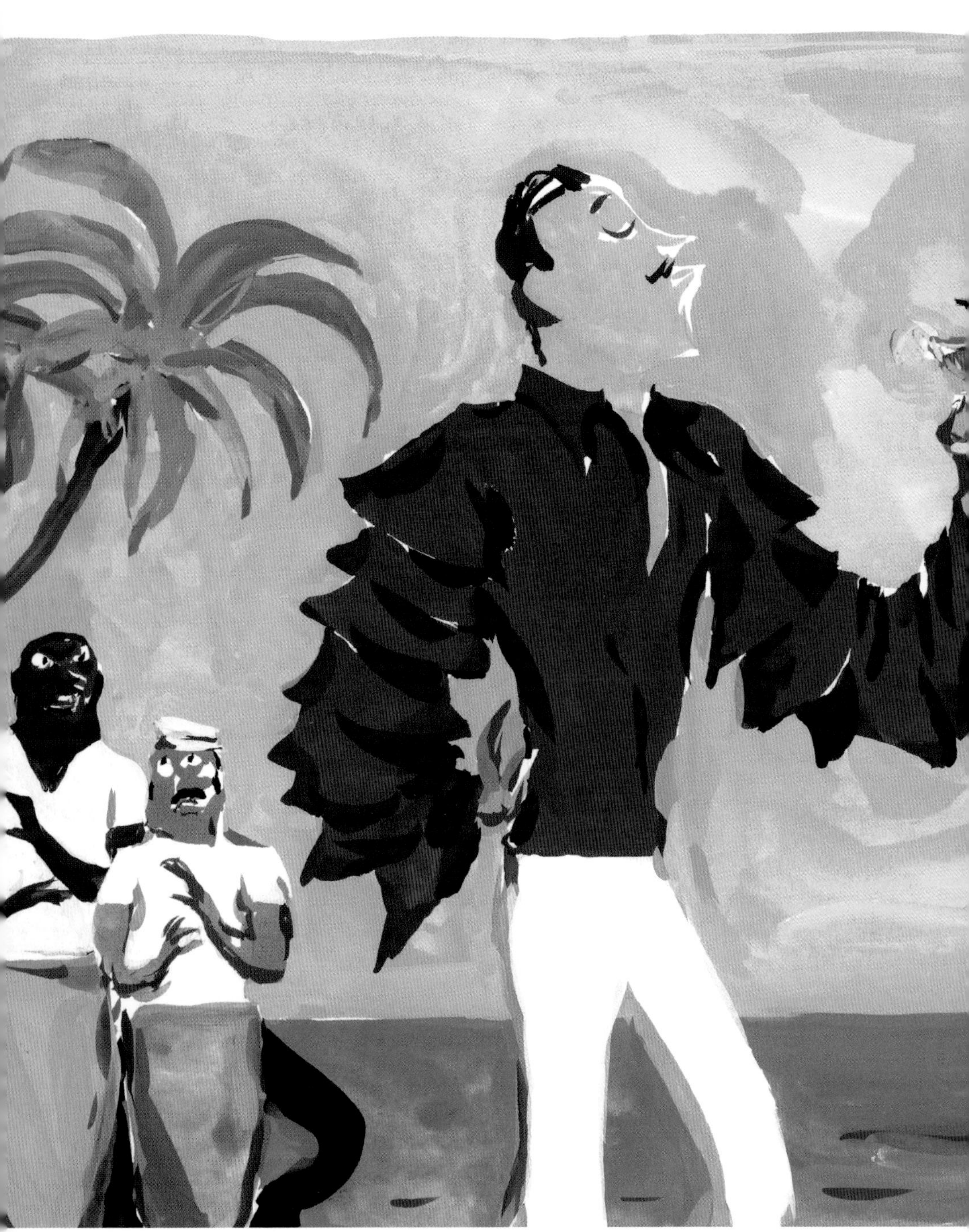

THROW CAUTION TO THE WIND

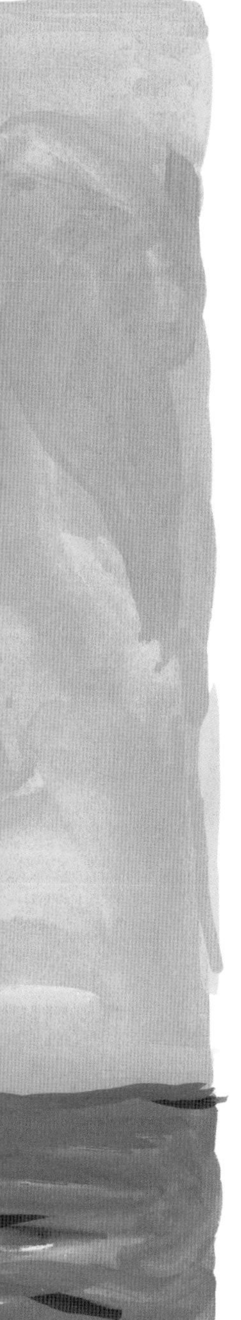

V — 001

WHEN CAN YOU WEAR A CALYPSO SHIRT?

This is a two-fold challenge. First—and probably the more difficult of the two—you need to find said shirt; doing so requires traveling to the Caribbean. Next, you have to find a suitable location to shake those ruffles out, just like one of those parrots that belong to elderly society women who meet every afternoon for tea and cakes. But why stop there? Should a shirt-maker get wind of this message, we would ask in no uncertain terms that he revive the fashion for calypso shirts, so that man may shine in all his glory—all day, every day. Until the Caribbean sun goes down.

V — 002

CAN YOU WEAR THE T-SHIRT IF YOU NEVER EVER LISTEN TO THE BAND?

Though 4G technology has enabled us to expand the breadth of our knowledge, we still claim the unalienable right to partial ignorance when it comes to personal style. Our garments are blazoned with the names of bands, computer games, TV show heroes, or basketball teams of which we know next to nothing—they're all fair game. What's the alternative? Go directly to jail. Do not pass go. Do not collect 200 dollars. Given the hit parade of favorite stars, if we sported names only of those we actually idolized, hundreds of thousands would be condemned to wear Michael Bolton hoodies. Fans of *Star Wars, Game of Thrones*, Kanye, and Candy Crush: don't hesitate to splash out on outfits in graphic prints that reflect the diametric opposite of your personal taste. Drawing from styles that differ from your own will give you the confidence you need to be dazzlingly resplendent.

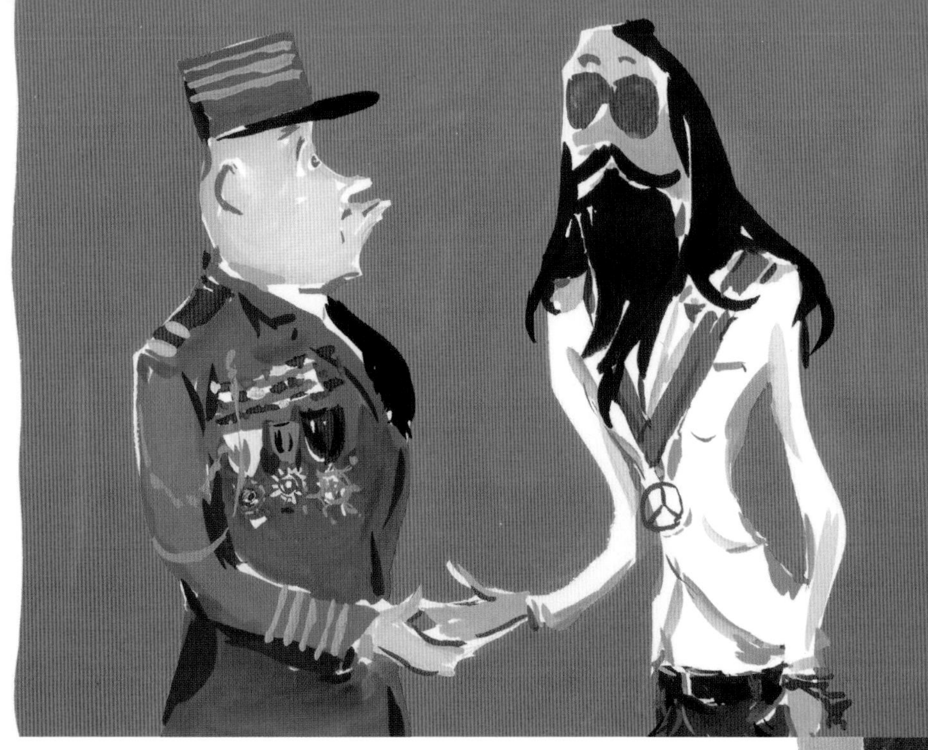

v —— 003

SHOULD MEN WEAR MEDALS?

A medal is designed to be a mark of distinction, awarded by an institution (a school, association, institute, or nation) to one of its illustrious members. Thus, wearing a medal is the mark of a hero. A large majority of dark-haired, extremely virile men have worn one—Cary Grant, Alain Delon, former French president Nicolas Sarkozy. Nowadays, everyone's a winner. We've forgotten what the medal was originally intended for, and postmodern society has perverted its use, turning it into a trophy for any average Joe. It is his mark of honor, his token of glory, worn as a sign of belonging to the herd, in total disregard of all the rest. The artist Bertrand Lavier said that there's a fine line between genius and bs. The same can be said about the superman and the moron. In conclusion, if you're going to wear a medal, wait until a big cheese decorates you.

v —— 004

HOW CAN YOU AVOID GETTING LOST IN THE SARTORIAL WOODS THIS WINTER?

What to wear? A plaid flannel shirt, mainly red. This is because, deep down, you are a lumberjack. Hiking boots made for rugged terrain. Long johns. A fine-knit sweater. Carry a thermos of coffee. And an old-fashioned suitcase, chicer than the kind with wheels. Finally, you've found the true colors of your lost flamboyance. Show them.

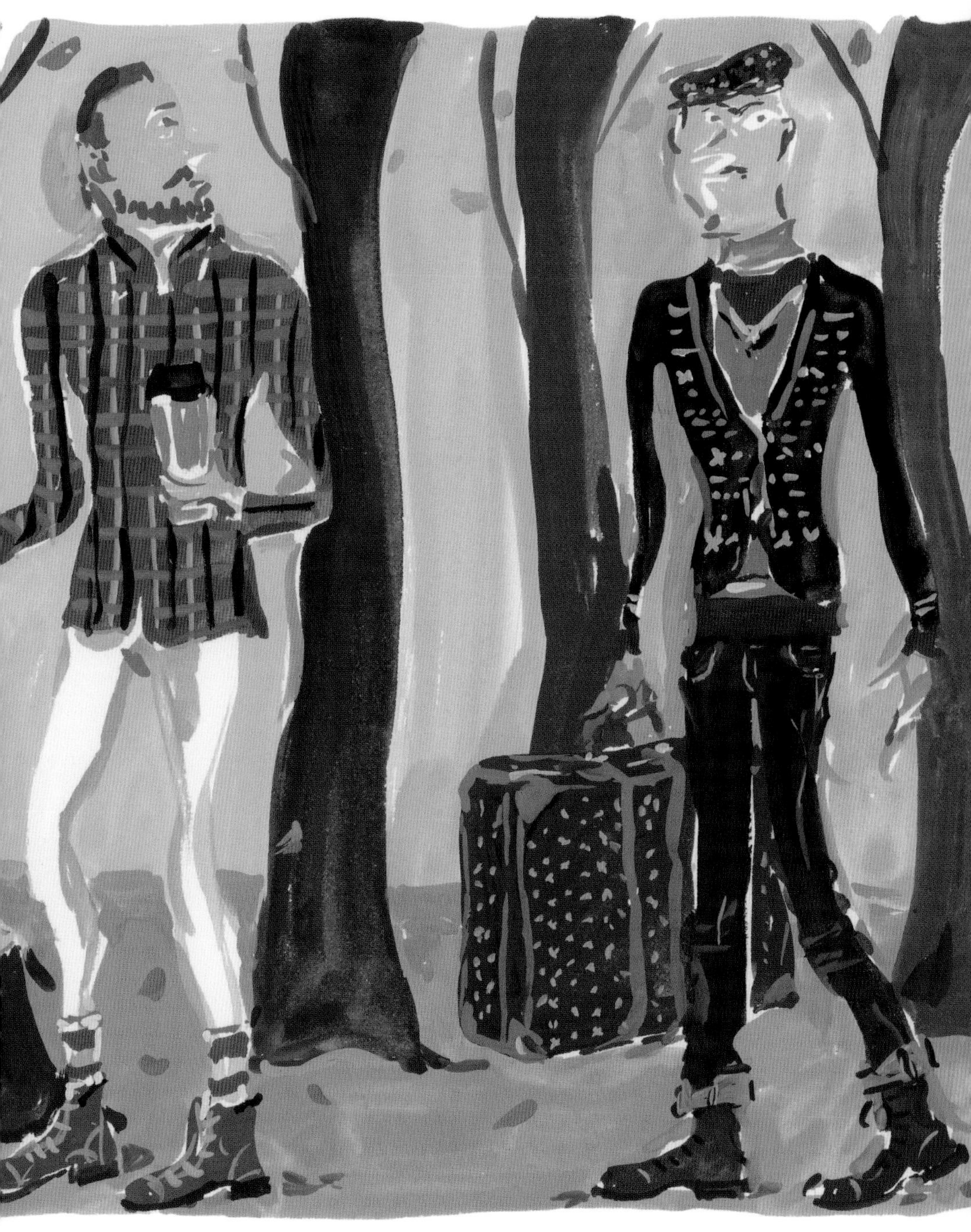

THROW CAUTION TO THE WIND

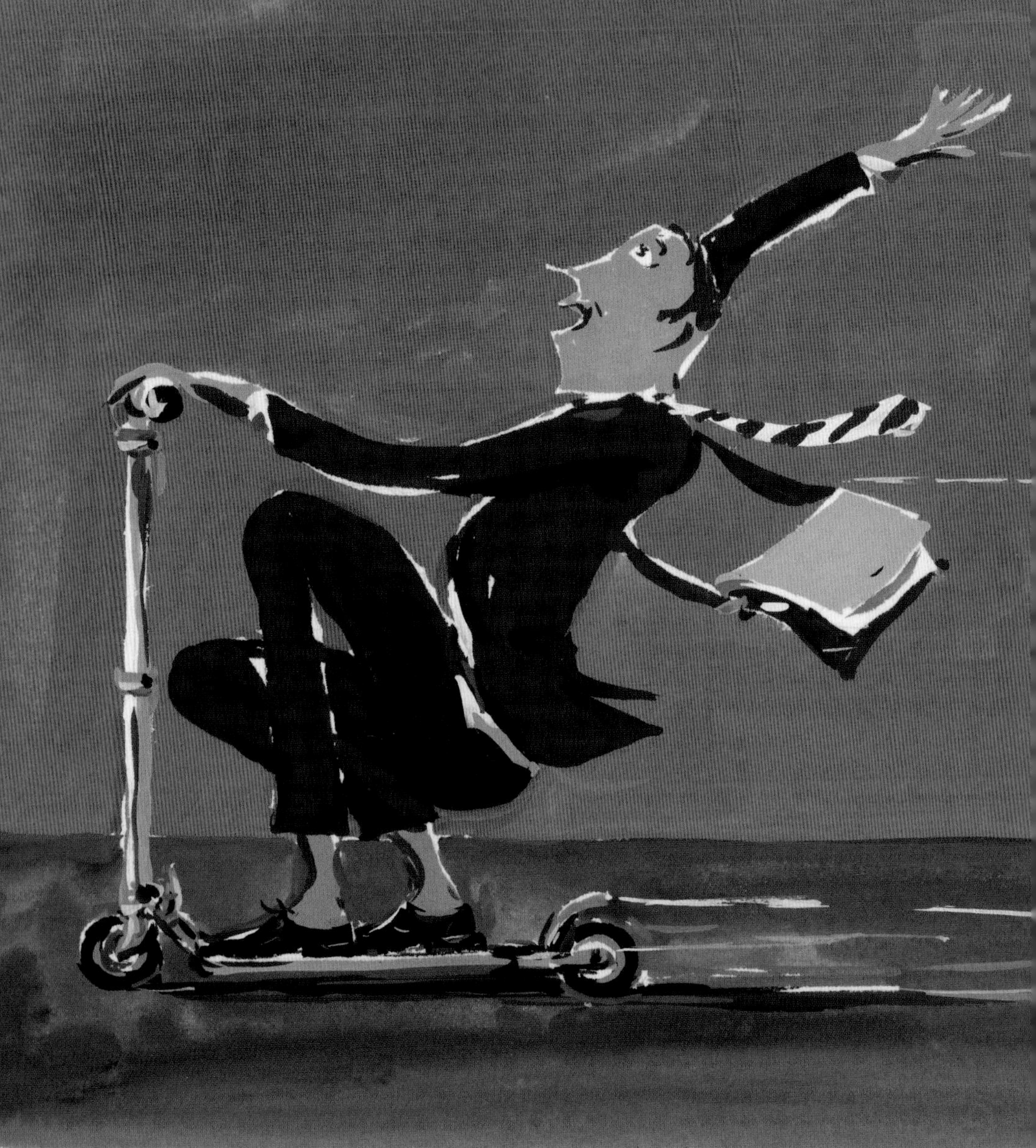

v —— 005

DO REAL MEN RIDE KICK SCOOTERS?

When our sidewalk-surfer friends take to the streets, the city turns into one big playground, with everyone whizzing around. Or that's what the ads are selling us. In reality, you scoot along, half squatting, like a madman, because your fear of being late for the bimonthly departmental meeting is worse than death itself. You have no idea how ridiculous you look, you're so focused on not running down some poor pedestrian. You should seriously consider carpooling or getting a bike.

v — 006

HOW CAN YOU TELL IF YOU'VE ARRIVED LATE FOR A DINNER?

If, when you arrive, your hosts are all seated in the living room, it means they've been waiting for you. On the other hand, if at the designated hour they are still sweeping up under the coffee table, you've arrived early. This is why you should arrive fifteen minutes after the stated time. A brief quarter of an hour, not half an hour. If you want to bring flowers, have them sent ahead of time.

v — 007

WHERE SHOULD YOU HIDE YOUR HANDKERCHIEF WHEN YOU HAVE A RUNNY NOSE?

In your pocket, a handkerchief turns into a dried-up ball or a sticky rag, so we suggest sliding it up your sleeve to the crook of your elbow. If you're wearing a sweater, you'll spend the winter with your sleeves pushed up. And if your nose is constantly running, you should probably seek professional advice.

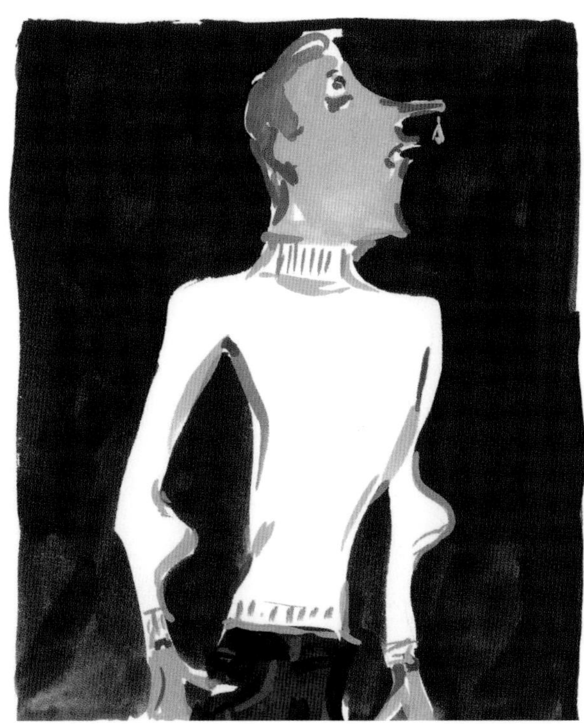

V —— 008

WHAT PET SHOULD YOU GET?

Over and above the love you have to bestow on a pet (careful, you might look ridiculous), the little beast has to meet the following criteria: smells good, doesn't lose its fur, shows independence but is subject to your natural authority and sensitive to your lifestyle, and is beautiful to behold at all times. This eliminates cats from the start, since they're more concerned with becoming Internet memes than making any effort to be appreciated in real life. Instead, make a comprehensive checklist of creatures that people would like to see at your place. We need not remind you that just one pet will suffice. If you're after something in a bowl, pick a seahorse, jellyfish, or octopus. For the adventurer: choose a scorpion, tarantula, snake, or iguana. To channel your inner Jack Sparrow, go for a parrot or a toucan (the less talkative the better). If you're a cynical epicurean, treat yourself to a peacock; the playboy should get a black panther. If you have the space, your menagerie can be enlarged to include horses or ponies. And don't forget birds of prey: they get rid of rodents and make a striking impression. And why not try a small flock of sheep, with you as shepherd? No goats, though—they can be devilish.

V —— 009

How should you dress for a Halloween party?

In a tux, to celebrate the romanticism of this Day of the Dead. Or as a canary, a toilet-paper mummy, or Austin Powers, if those are the only costumes you have. Remember, all you really have to do is play the game. Too many parties are ruined because of a playlist battle or YouTube video competition. Make your mark and dress however you want; even if you're way off target, it'll put you in high spirits and show that, like a typical Parisian, you're bloody-minded. Just a drop.

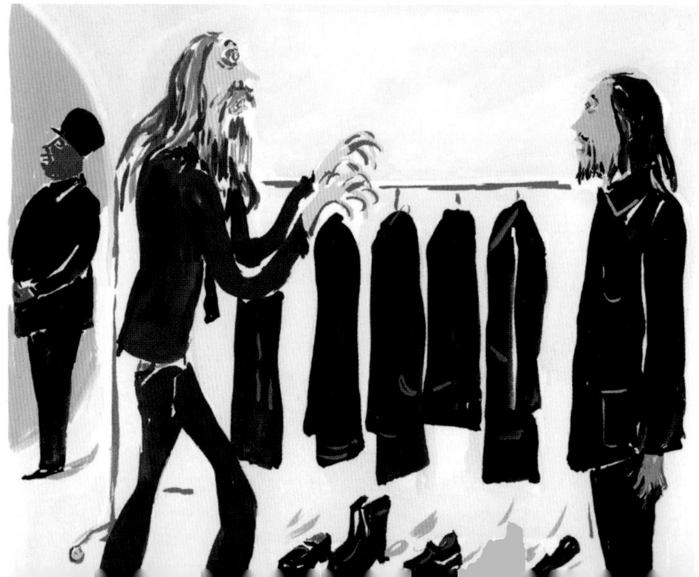

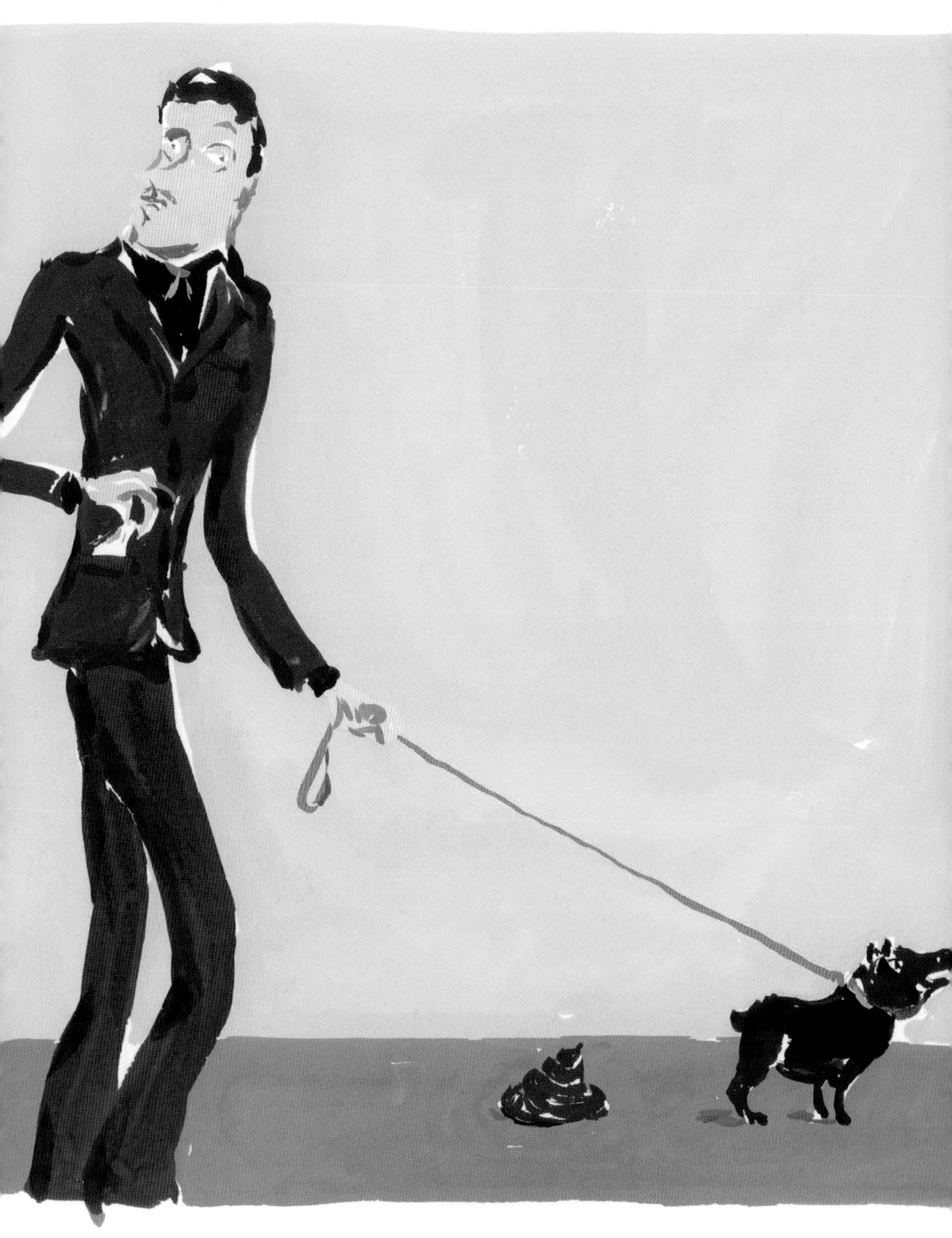

THROW CAUTION TO THE WIND

V — 010

IS IT TIME FOR A POCKET SQUARE COMEBACK?

The pocket square has been out of style for quite some time—maybe it just seemed too fussy and so it fell out of favor. But the pendulum of fashion swings back and forth between an image of timelessness and a generational vision of masculine elegance. A pocket square does have its uses: for a man who is anxious about a less-than-toned waist, it draws the eyes up, toward the shoulders (and double chin). Even so, today it is going through a bad spell, since no one, not even those old dandies who are *so* last century, wants to hear about it. Washed, folded, and put away, it is patiently waiting to come out of its enforced hibernation.

V — 011

WHAT'S THE NEW KILT?

Brought up on a diet of grunge, you have probably noticed that tying your lumberjack shirt around your waist recalls the traditional clothing of Scottish warriors. Now that you are aware of the analogy, you have a wonderful excuse to do the same.

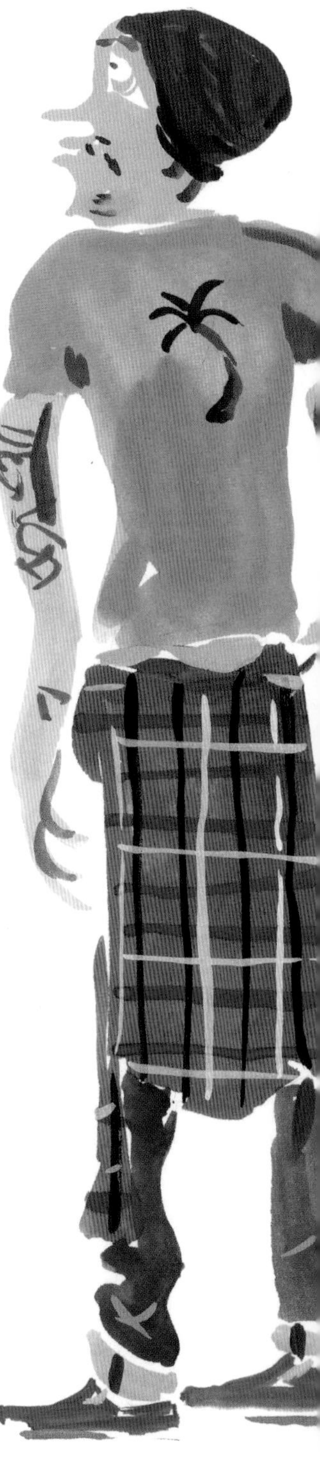

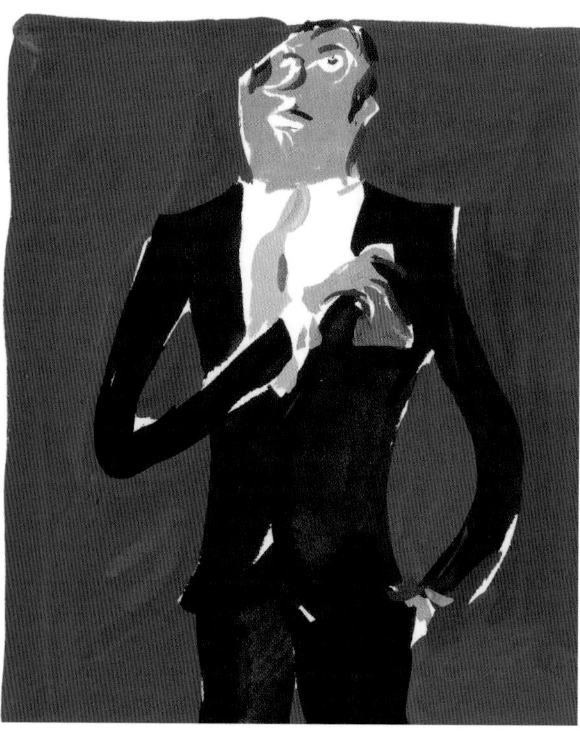

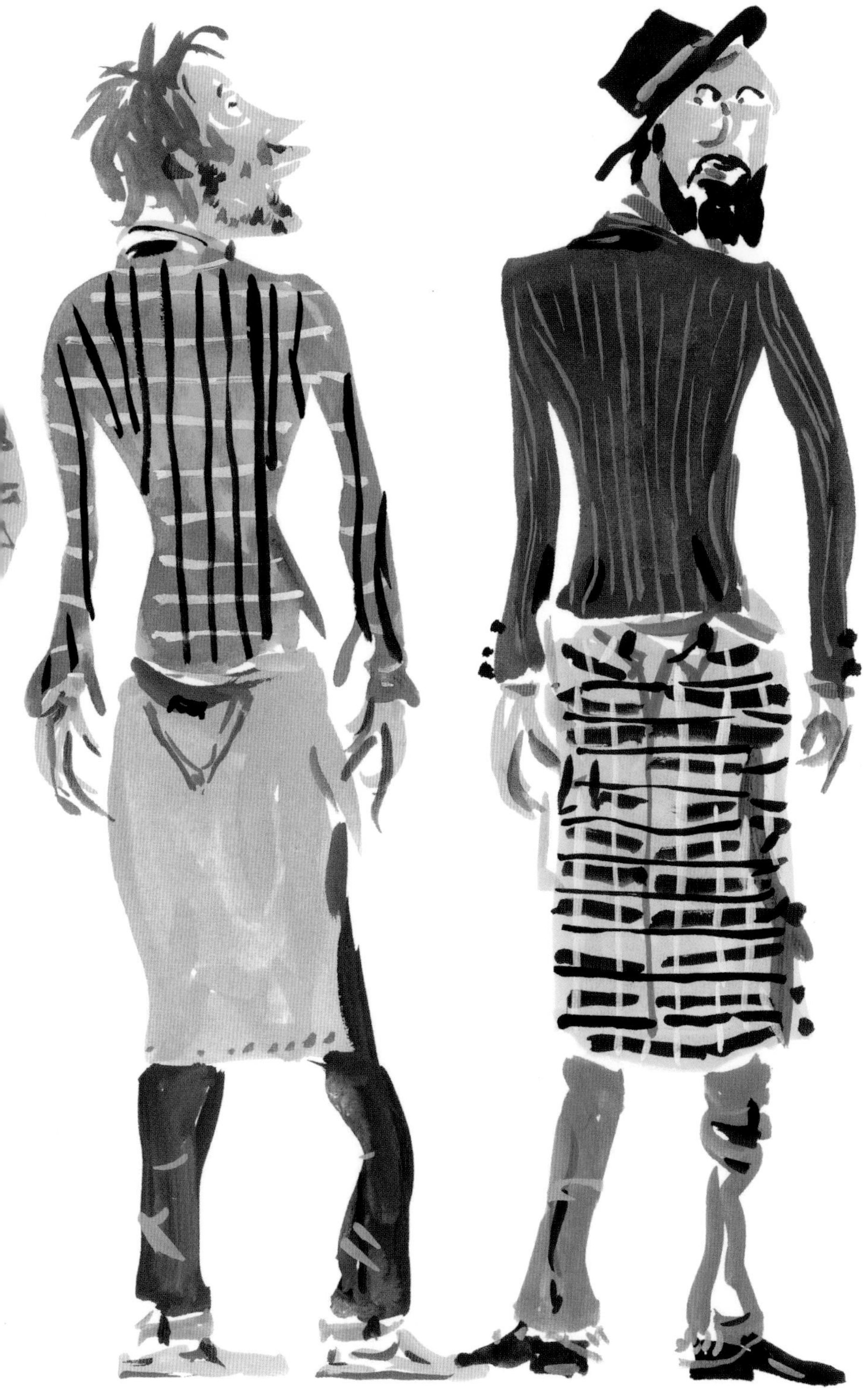

THROW CAUTION TO THE WIND

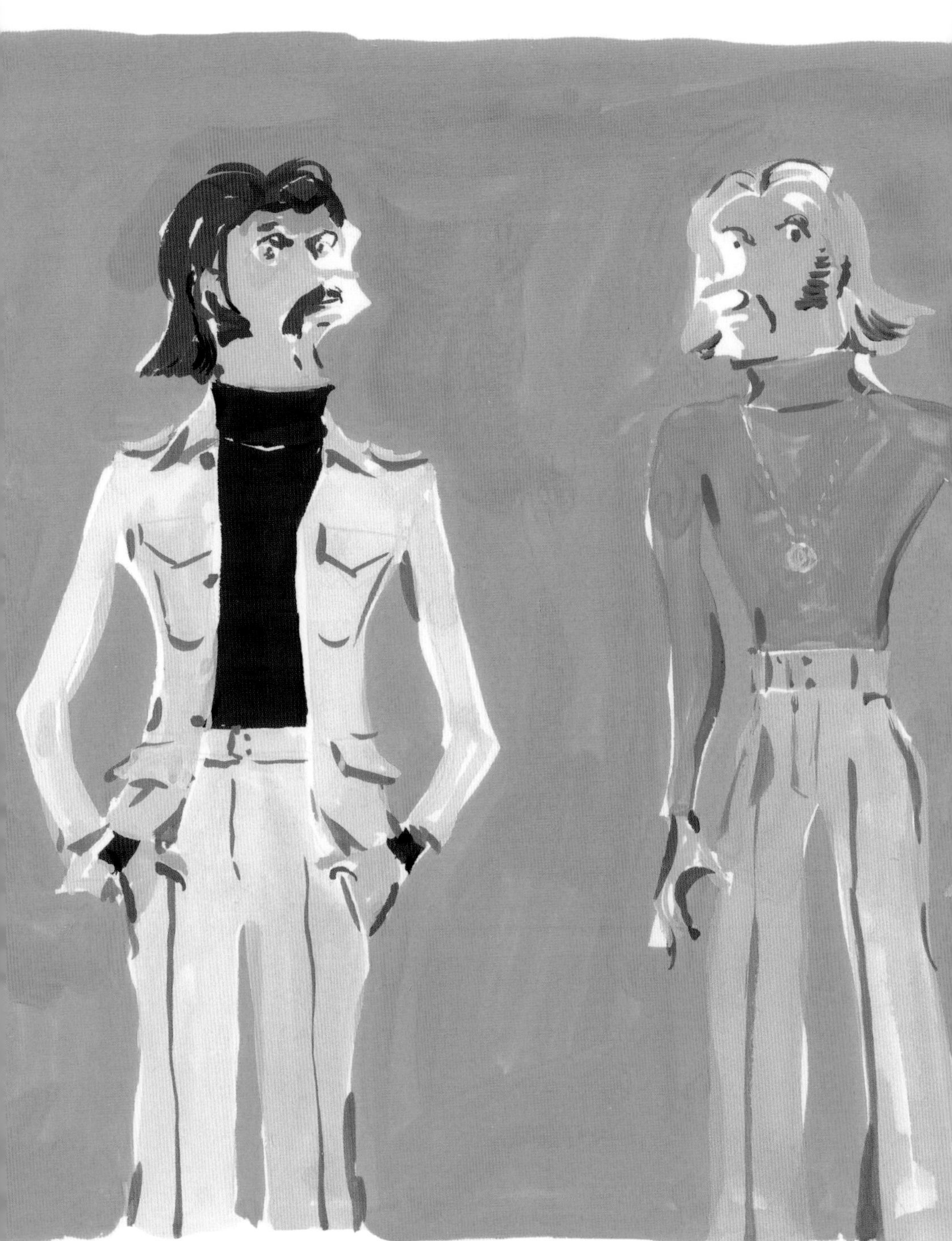

THROW CAUTION TO THE WIND

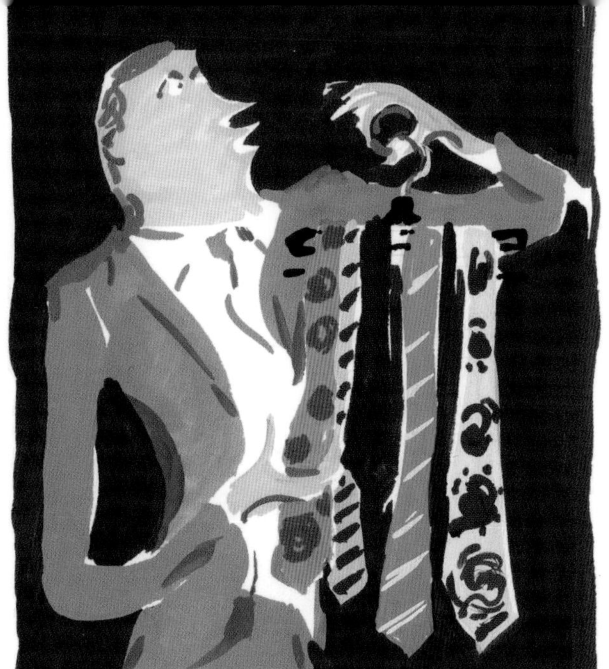

v —— 012

WHY ON EARTH WOULD YOU HANG UP YOUR NECKTIES?

The French actor Jean-Paul Belmondo displayed his love of neckties in the film *Ho!,* which came out in 1968 (music lovers may remember the soundtrack by François de Roubaix). In the film, directed by Robert Enrico, Public Enemy Number One collects neckties, carefully stored away with the help of a special rack. At one point, he leaves his hideout to buy an incredible tie made of coconut fiber. Back home, he flips through his tie collection with incredible speed. For this very reason, we authorize the purchase of such a storage system. The usual solution of suspending them on a hanger is very inconvenient, as they slip off onto the floor every time you touch them. The modern man must therefore meet the challenge of finding a rack for them (a sliding one if possible, so the ties can be admired in natural light), or else he must roll them up so they can be slipped into small yet immensely convenient compartments in his drawer.

v —— 013

SHOULD YOU TUCK IN YOUR SWEATER?

Don't be ashamed of asking an idiotic question if you don't know the answer. As a fan of the fashion shows, you'll have seen dozens of models wearing their sweaters tucked in. We wish to dissuade you from copying them. A model's main aim, considering the economic stake he represents, is to display clearly what he is wearing, which includes the belt. This—let's be realistic here—is not exactly the case with you.

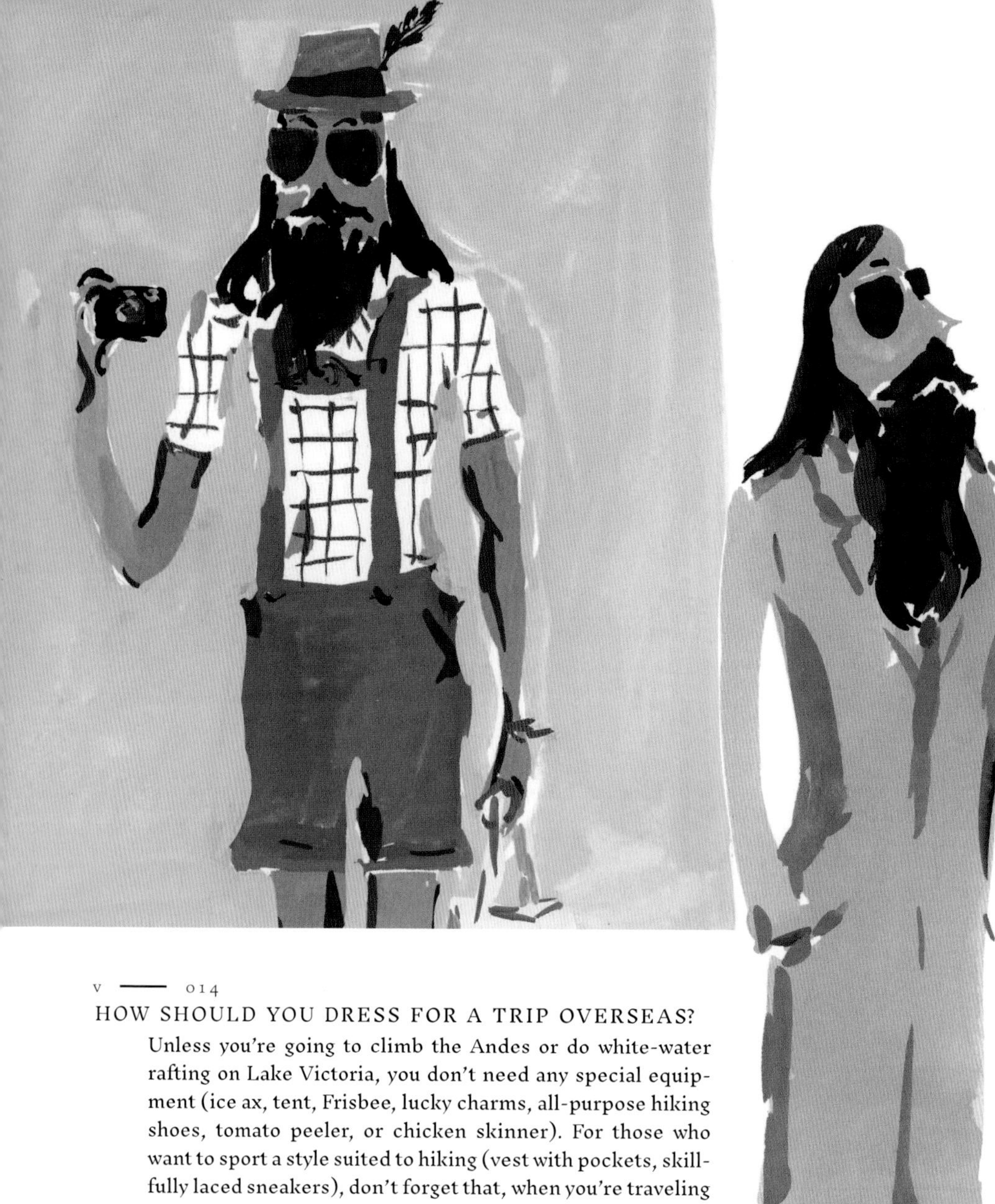

V —— 014

HOW SHOULD YOU DRESS FOR A TRIP OVERSEAS?

Unless you're going to climb the Andes or do white-water rafting on Lake Victoria, you don't need any special equipment (ice ax, tent, Frisbee, lucky charms, all-purpose hiking shoes, tomato peeler, or chicken skinner). For those who want to sport a style suited to hiking (vest with pockets, skillfully laced sneakers), don't forget that, when you're traveling in foreign lands, people are observing you. You have a reputation to uphold, so exercise a little discipline and be your nation's style ambassador.

V —— 015

SHOULD YOU TAKE OFF YOUR GLASSES WHEN YOU KISS SOMEBODY ON THE CHEEK?

There's no practical reason to remove them, unless you head-butt your friends to say hello or you're the only one wearing sunglasses. Just be careful you and the other person don't bump into each other. Ultimately, however, taking off your glasses is the suave thing to do.

V —— 016

WILL A CAMEL-COLORED COAT MAKE IT THROUGH THE WINTER TUNDRA?

What a poetic question. The camel coat is elegant but doesn't actually suit many people. We find it annoying and kind of ugly. Since it's pale, it has to stay impeccably clean, and the wearer must always be well turned out. This pristine look isn't our thing: it reminds us of the kid at school who wouldn't go out to play in case he got dirty. The camel-colored coat is typically worn by the realtor that this kid became, because he never took any risks in life. It's also the overcoat favored by the father-in-law with the veneer smile. Go for (yet) another more conventional color.

V —— 017

Should we stop wearing fur-trimmed hoods?

Yes. That furry mane around your head ends up being a real headache. But, alas, it's pretty much unavoidable, with the ugly clothing brigade out in force.

V —— 018

WHY DO SOME EUROPEAN LUXURY HOTELS RING A BELL AT SIX O'CLOCK IN THE MORNING?

This clever device allows absent-minded guests who mistakenly found themselves in the wrong room to get back to their own before sunrise.

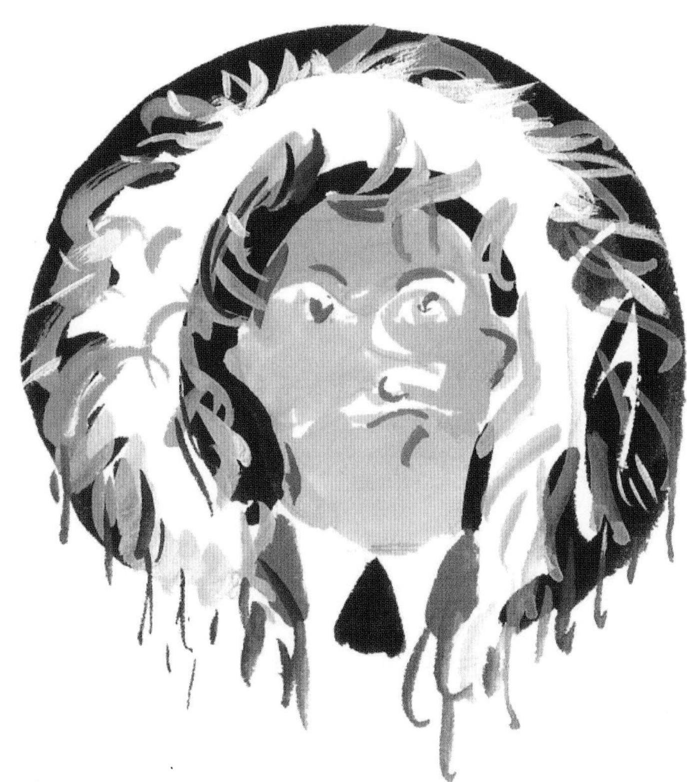

V —— 019

HOW CAN YOU LOOK SUAVE WHEN TAKING A TOKE?

It's not like it happens every day, but one of your artist friends passes you a recreational cigarette that he is holding up vertically by the filter. With your index and middle fingers, make the victory sign and take it. Tilt your head back slightly when taking a drag, inhaling slowly so that the tip retains an intriguing color. Blow the smoke out of your nose right away as you move your head back to its usual position. Remain silent, without giving the impression you're involved in some kind of pagan rite. Join the conversation again as soon as your voice no longer sounds pinched due to the smoke in your lungs.

V —— 020

IS IT OK TO SPLASH AROUND WITH A MASK AND SNORKEL?

If you are more coordinated on land than in water, we're talking to you. You arrive at the beach, or your favorite manmade lake, with your charming raffia basket. Inside there is a veritable arsenal, to be handled with care. First up, the flippers: they allow you to perform the butterfly stroke like a god. But is it worth keeping up the effort when no one is watching you from the shore? And did you forget that you have to slip them on when you're in the water, while either standing or half-floating? Then there's the mask and snorkel. Over the age of fifteen, a passion for inspecting the underwater world at a depth of seven feet is no longer acceptable. To win us over, you'll need an inflatable boat, cylinders, and an early-morning foray into the deep.

V —— 021

CAN YOU WEAR SHORTS TO A BEACHSIDE RESTAURANT?

After showering, resting, and slathering on the after-sun cream, some men wear pants to make sure they are offered a complimentary limoncello at that little pizzeria on the harbor suggested by TripAdvisor. You, however, with your skin still tight from the sea salt and your shorts still damp from the last swim at sundown, may not smell like Irish Spring Men's Body Wash, but you are fully experiencing the joys of letting go while on vacation. To hell with the mosquitoes, adventure calls to guide you through your week off.

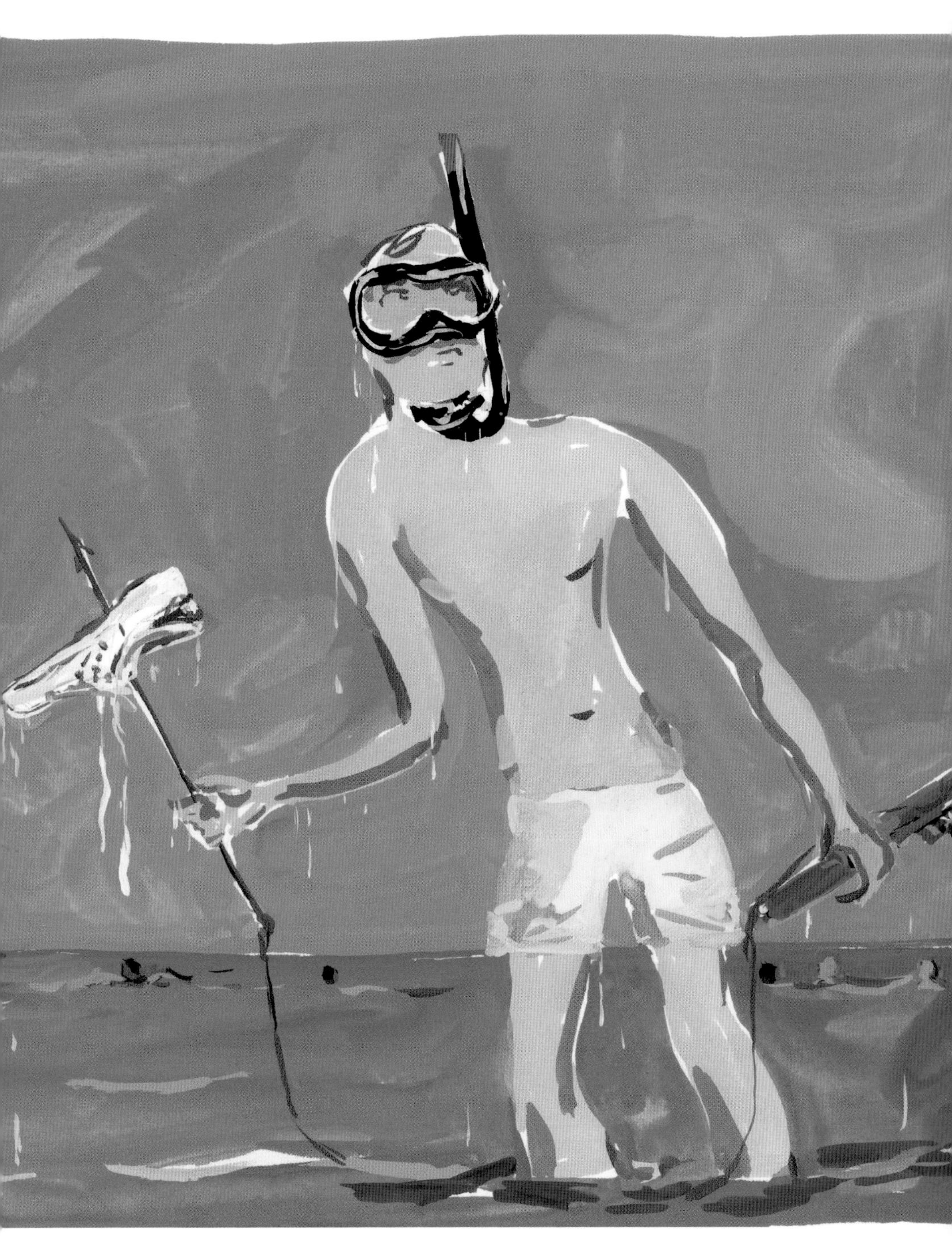

THROW CAUTION TO THE WIND

CXIV

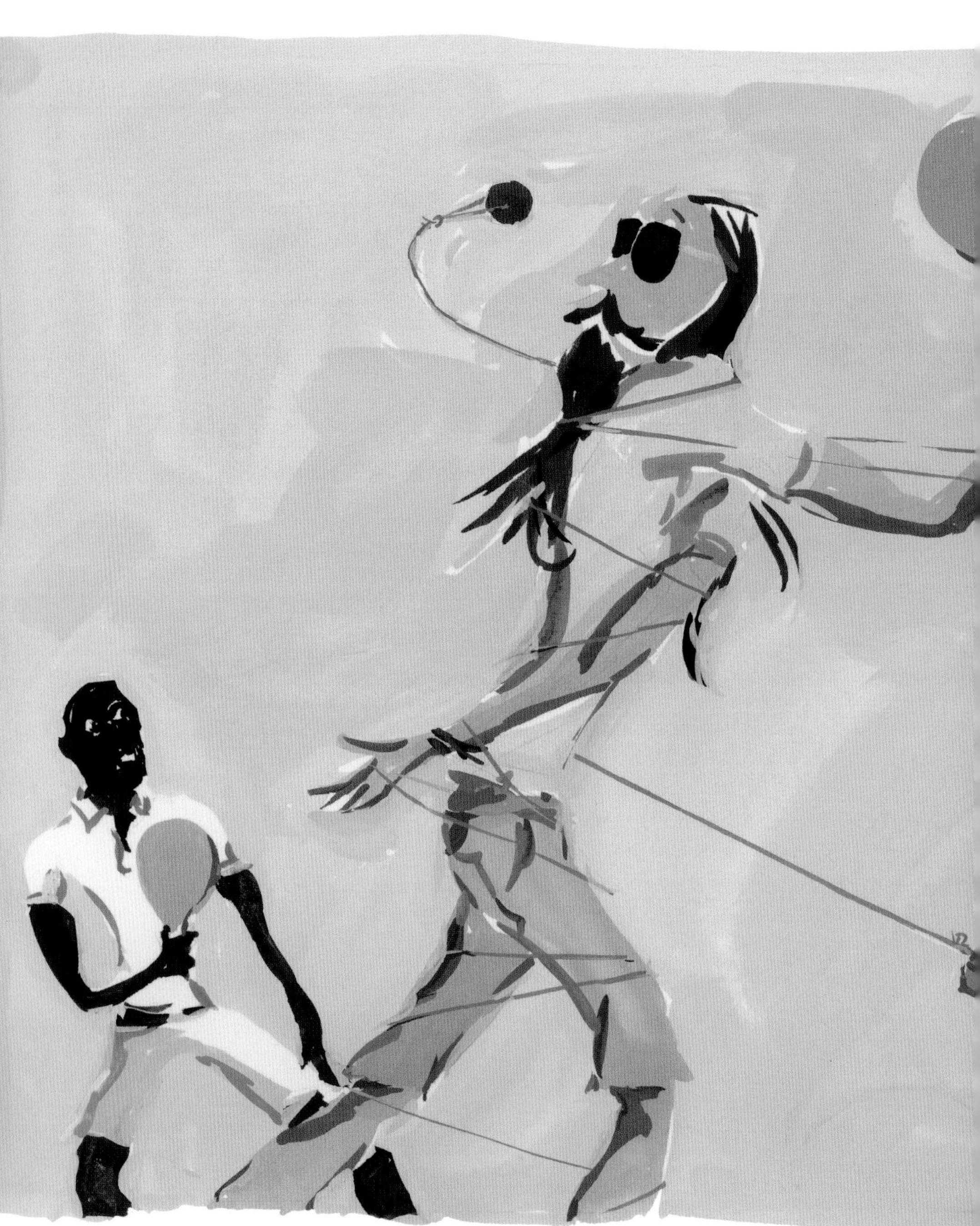

THROW CAUTION TO THE WIND

v —— 022

WHICH SPORT WILL BE ON TREND THIS SUMMER?

After the sensational and unexpected comeback of *pétanque* in France this past decade, it is high time we brought a more athletic sport back from oblivion. We totally love the idea of digging out our old paddle ball set from the garage. That's because this racket sport, which originated in the Basque country in the interwar years, can be played alone or in a group, almost anywhere and in any clothes (except a tux), even while having an aperitif. Otherwise, there is backgammon, another of our favorite games, but it's somewhat lacking in elastic-pinging fun.

v —— 023

HOW CAN YOU KEEP A TRAIN CAR TO YOURSELF?

You have no idea how much we like it when you break the rules. When it comes to repelling others, there is no better invention than hard-boiled eggs, greek gyro, or hamburgers.

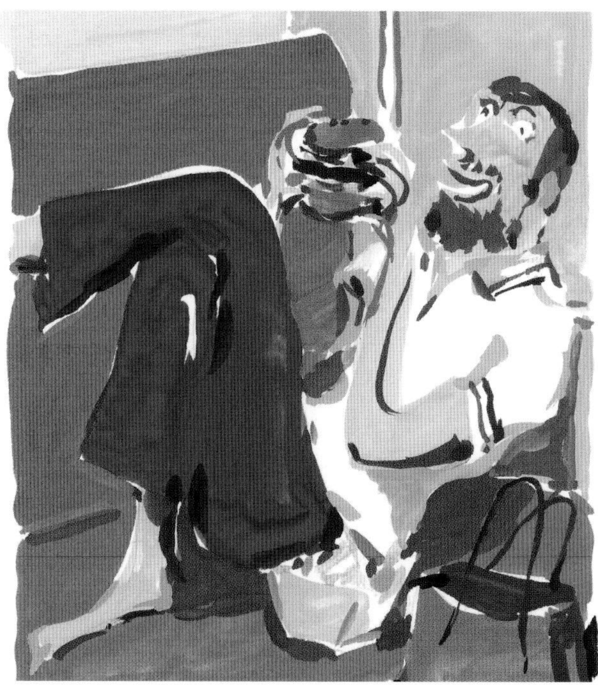

V —— 024

WHAT'S THE BEST WAY TO DRY AN UMBRELLA?

Paul Frey, cofounder of the brand Kumo—a French maker of artist-designed umbrellas—immediately came to our rescue: "To dry an umbrella, keep it open, with the fabric stretched, for the same reasons as for clothes or socks: because the dampness can damage the fabric where it's folded. Also, be careful not to let the umbrella dry too close to a source of heat. Dry it at room temperature for best results." This should make your parquet floor happy.

V —— 025

WHAT'S THE ONE PIECE OF CLOTHING THAT EVERY PERFECT GENTLEMAN NEEDS?

You guessed it—a cape! Used and abused by French gendarmes back in the 1940s, worn to dazzling effect by all self-respecting superheroes, it is now making a quiet comeback. A cape should fall to the mid-thigh, never higher (the Little Red Riding Hood effect), never lower (Casanova, or Dracula).

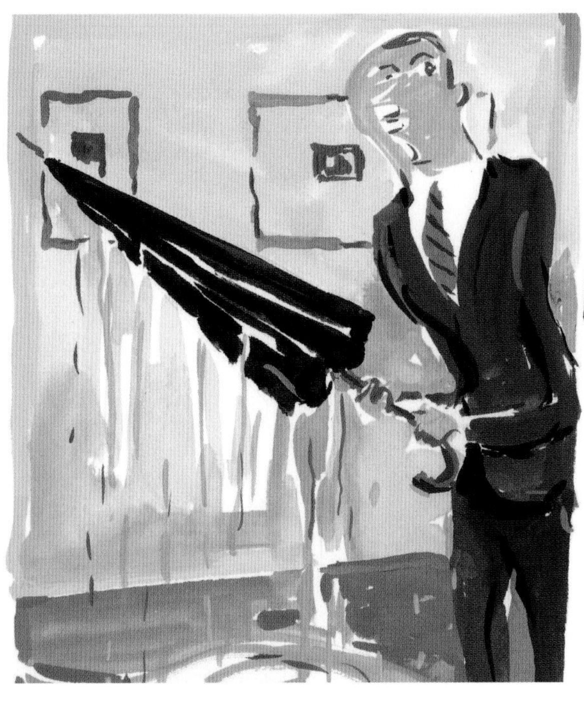

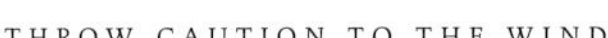

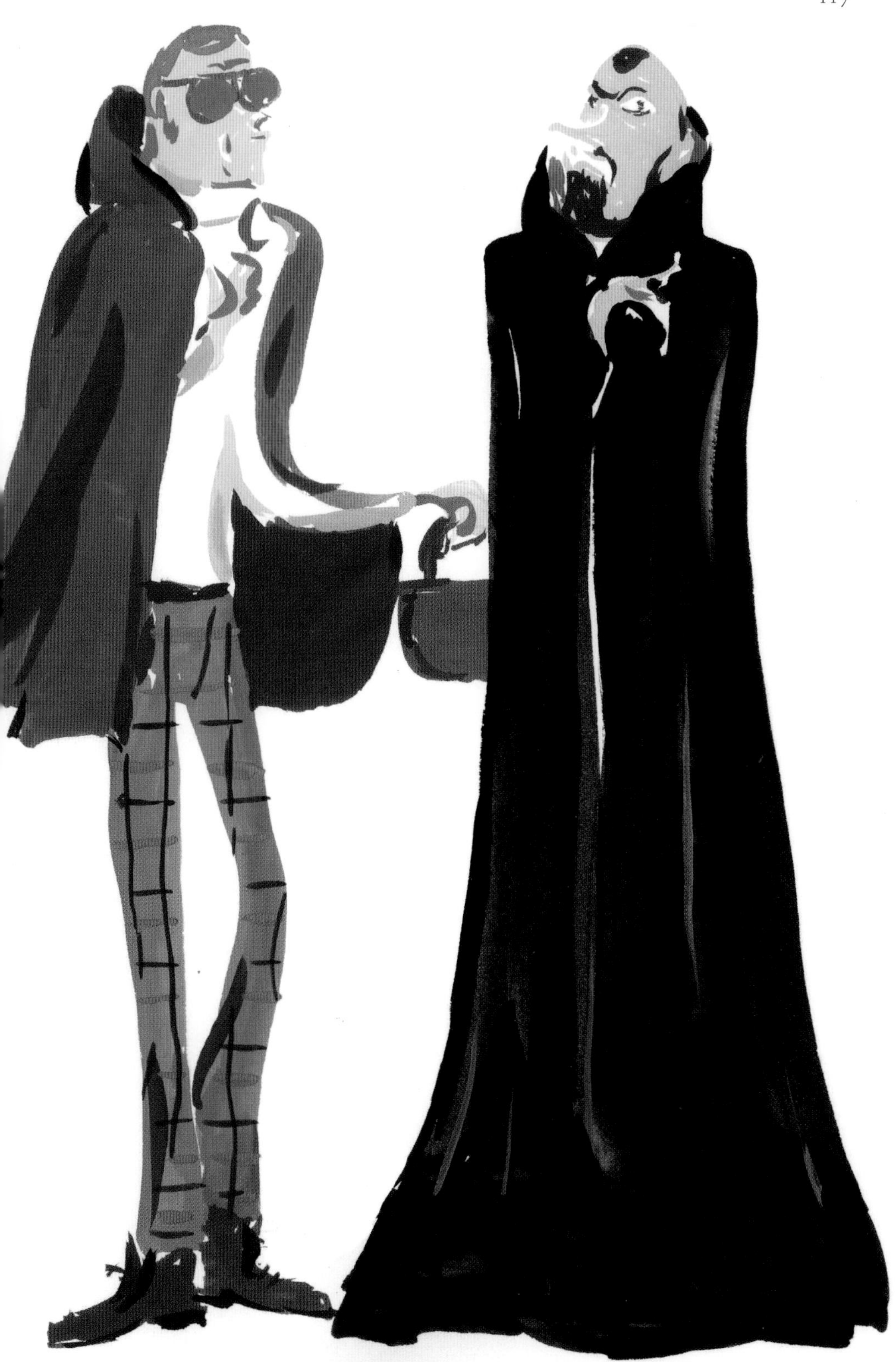

v —— 026

HOW CAN YOU LOOK LIKE A BOSS IN GRAND THEFT AUTO V?

There's nothing simpler, my friends. Of the three characters, choose the sociopath, Trevor Philips. When the game starts, you'll see him, sallow skinned, in a repulsive T-shirt. Let him commit a few larcenies. He loves that. Then take him to the hairdresser and ask for a long cut (it can be done), so that his receding hairline goes as far as his exploits. Win some money, beat up a few innocent passersby, then take him for a stroll in the luxury stores. A black tux awaits him at Ponsonbys on Portola Drive. Head to Binco, a thrift store, find a trucker's cap, and there you have it. Steal a private jet from the airport and take a trip through this fantasy world while flicking through radio stations.

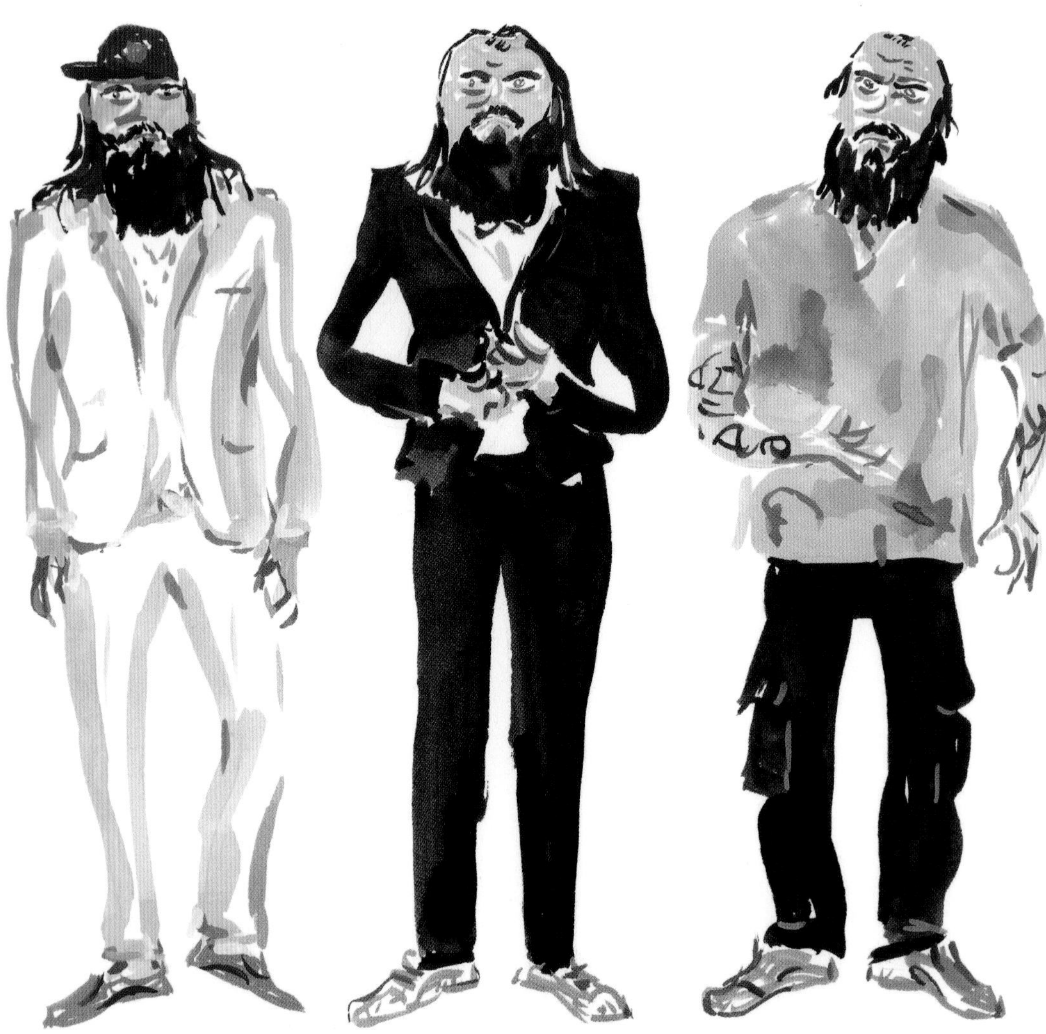

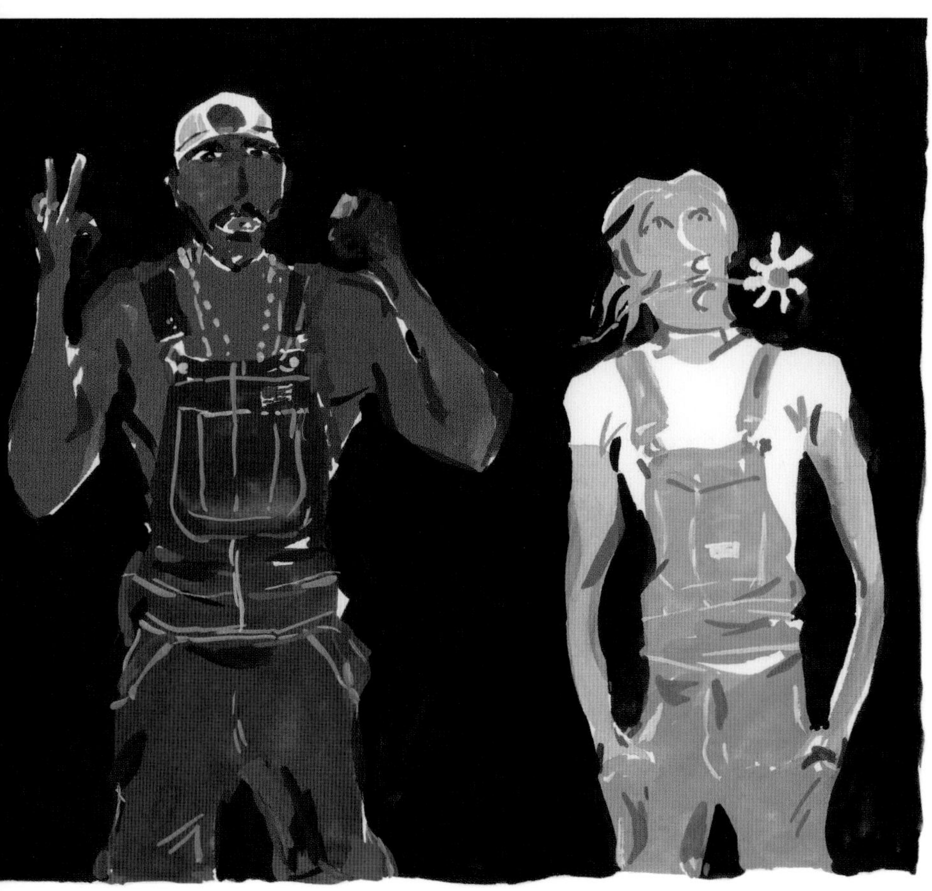

V —— 027

WHAT'S THE BEST WAY TO WEAR OVERALLS?

There's farmer style and there's street style. If you're big and fat, you can do the farmer look; blond and young, go for Brad Pitt in the early 1990s. And when you're cool (and black), you can rock this garment Tupac-style. Though with all due respect to the late author of "California Love," his attire wasn't exactly in the best of taste. So what can we expect from a major comeback of this timeless garb, unanimously celebrated by fashionistas? Although the style references make fashion sense, let's keep a gentlemanly maxim in mind, one that, although rarely followed these days, can be applied to any situation, from the most confusing to the most embarrassing: "Women and children first."

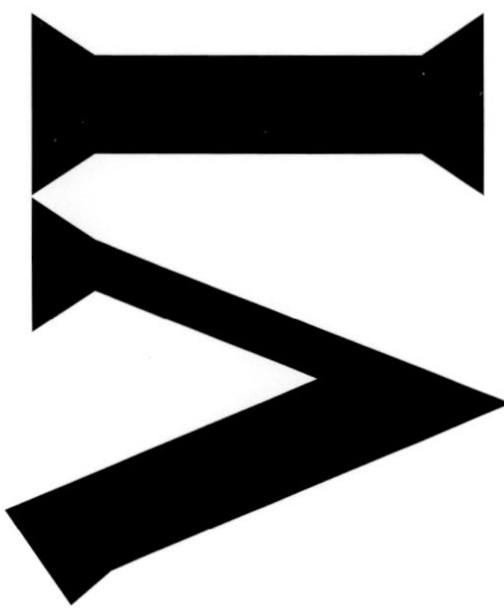

LIVE WITH YOUR OWN

VI —— 001 › VI —— 021

How should you conduct yourself on the telephone? • Should you go for #@!& bangs? • Why are France's leading literary luminaries often mistaken for matadors? • Do you have to look good when you exercise? • What's the best way to offer someone a breath freshener? • What's with blue bloods and loud colors? • How can you be a suave metalhead? • What's a guido? • What's the best way to deal with a hangover? • How should you dress when you're with people cooler than you? • Should you resist the Bowie hype? • How can you (more*

(BAD) TASTE

or less) pull off wearing suspenders? • Should you go for a floral print? • Can you keep your helmet on at the bakery? • Where does the chinstrap beard come from? • Is it ok to wear a Russian hat in an elevator? • What's the verdict on sneakers with flashing soles? • Are pre-tied bow ties acceptable? • Why cut off your sweatshirt at the elbows? • Which hair issues are much ado about nothing? • Should you "werk it" with your eyebrows?

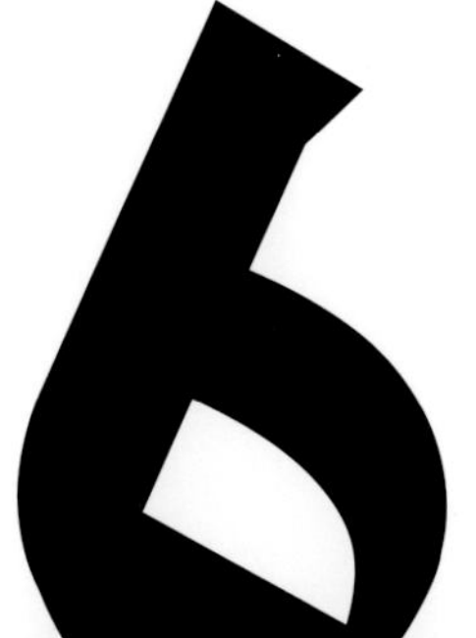

CHAPTER SIX

VI —— 001

HOW SHOULD YOU CONDUCT YOURSELF ON THE TELEPHONE?

The powers that be should give free rein to the following seven commandments:
1. Always call back. As soon as possible. Except those who are a real pain in the neck.
2. Stay discreet. Pick a ringtone with a simple melody, keep the volume low, and have your conversations at a distance from others. Your telephone should never be visible on the table, except at the office.
3. Stay courteous. The caller should end the conversation.
4. Abstain. Text messages and emails should not intrude on a conversation in person without permission from the person you are talking to.
5. Be decent. Never discuss the size of your phone bills or the performance of your device—subjects that impress you alone.
6. Stay suave. Put the telephone away in the inside pocket of your jacket or back pocket of your jeans.
7. Look for your telephone before you say you've lost it. And don't enlist an army to help you find it.

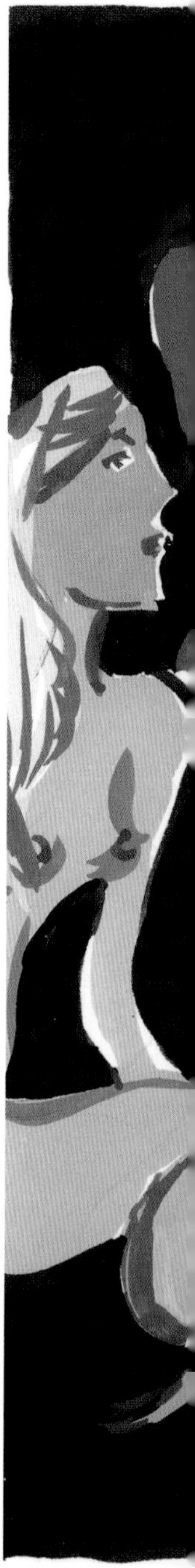

VI —— 002

SHOULD YOU GO FOR #@!&* BANGS?

The young male has always used his hair to broadcast his disdain for parental authority, allowing his unkempt locks to fall in his eyes, all the better to convey "whatevs." A few years later—older now, with a helmet hanging from his elbow—there he is, diligently making skinny lattes and soya decaf cappucinos with the tousled hair of a guy who has just leapt out of bed and onto his motor scooter. It goes without saying that it is strictly forbidden for you to be so cavalier with your disheveled esthetic.

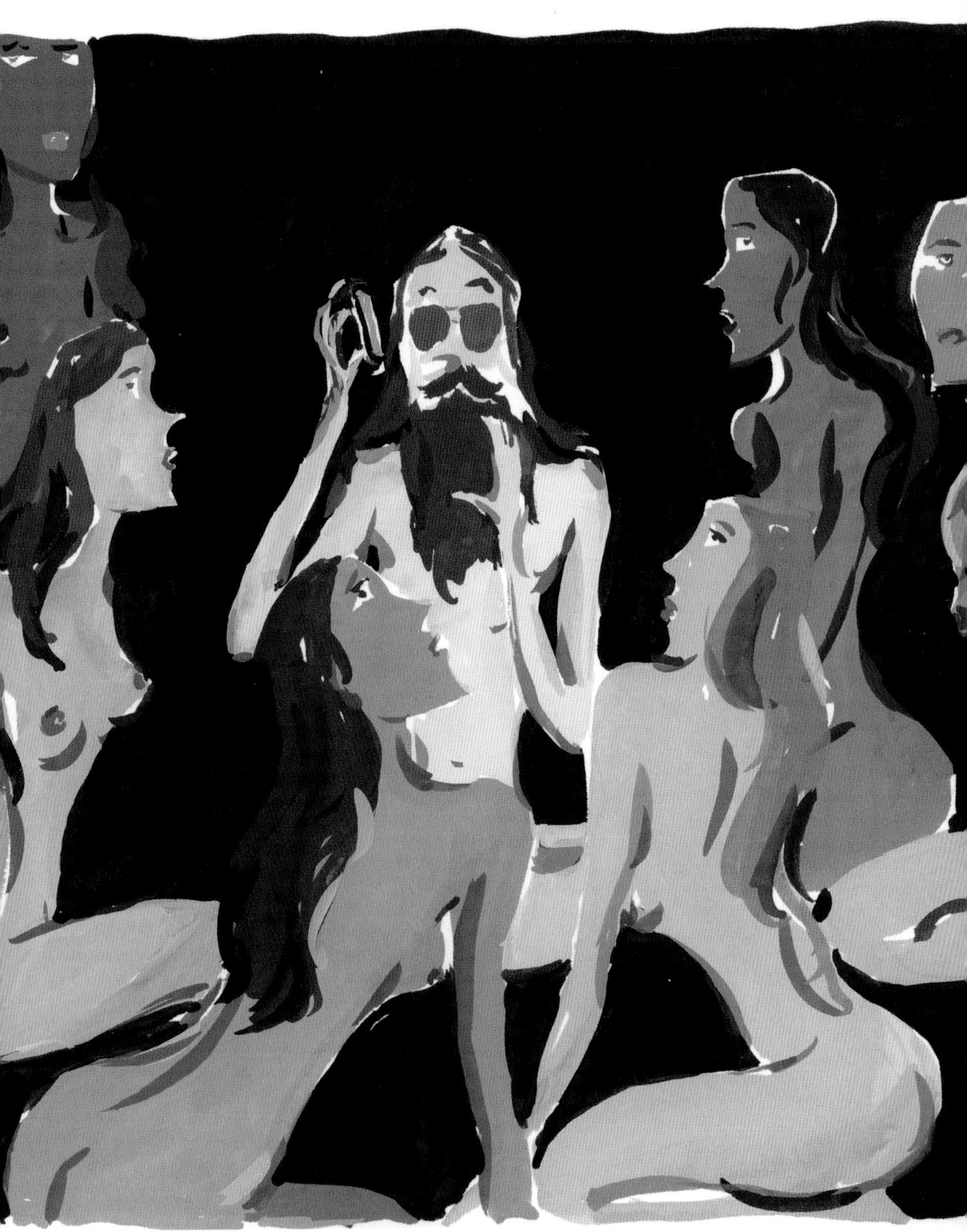

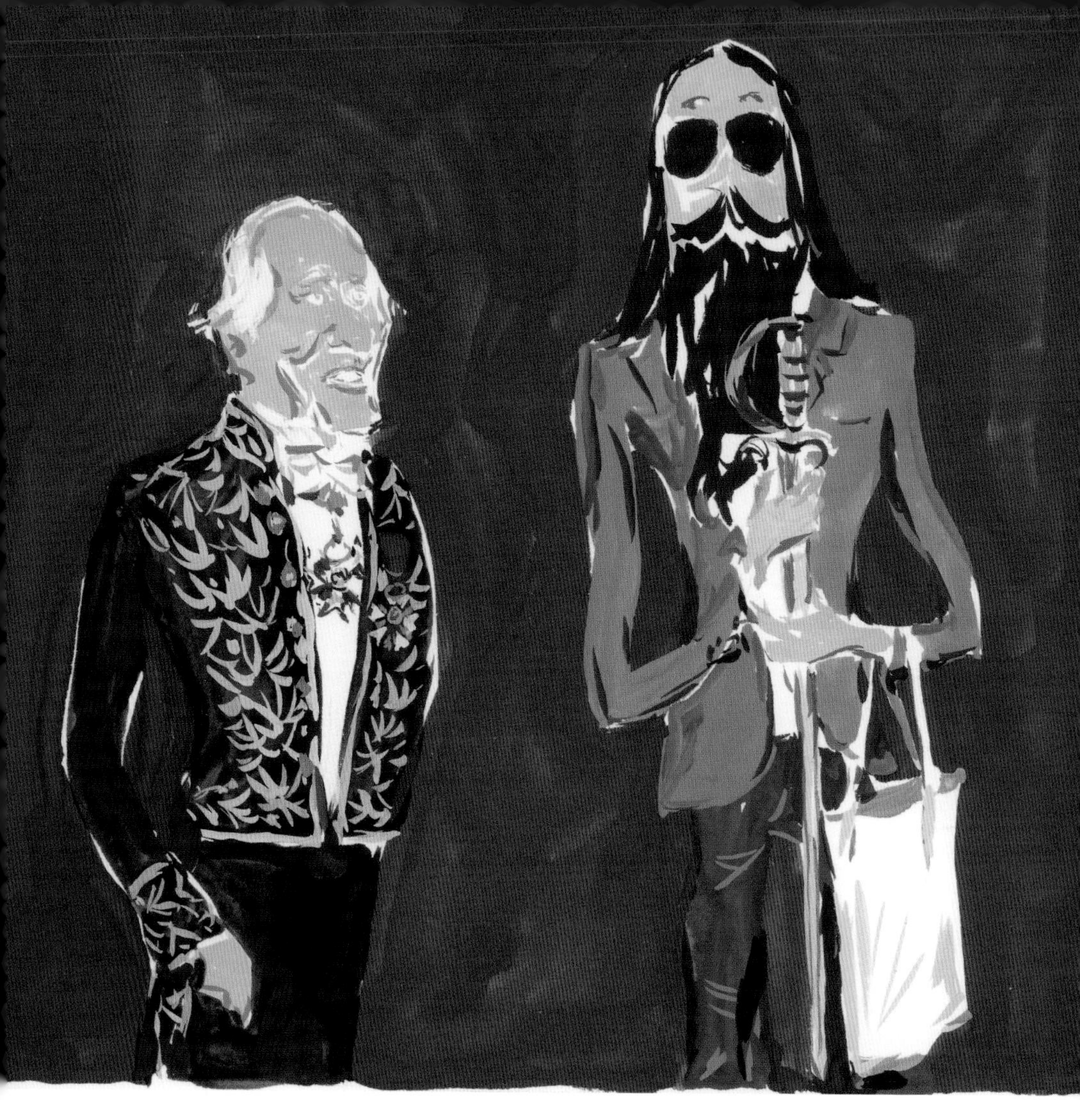

VI —— 003

WHY ARE FRANCE'S LEADING LITERARY LUMINARIES OFTEN MISTAKEN FOR MATADORS?

The honorable Académie Française—the French Academy—was established in 1635 by Cardinal de Richelieu to safeguard the French language. Its forty members comprise an exclusive group. They sport official attire: a jacket embroidered with an olive-leaf motif, pants trimmed with a stripe down the side, white vest, white shirt, bow tie, cape, three-cornered hat, and sword. This is the strict minimum, to which each member adds an individual twist depending on his or her own official decorations. The cost is borne by the French Academy member, but generous donors have been known to help finance the sword. The outfit's resemblance to the bullfighter costume is remarkable, and the (aging) members are no less bloodthirsty when it comes to protecting the French language from dilution by foreign words.

VI —— 004

DO YOU HAVE TO LOOK GOOD WHEN YOU EXERCISE?

The more you frequent places where exercise machines, mirrors, and mats have replaced classic training infrastructure (running tracks, sports fields, rings, judo mats, climbing walls), the greater the pressure to look good. A jogger or badminton player in a natural setting will be more easily forgiven for wearing a shapeless T-shirt, tearaway athletic pants, and argyle socks, whereas the exerciser who neglects to combine their cropped pants with a pair of the very latest sneakers will be hounded out of zumba class. The velour tracksuit, made popular by a German manufacturer, remains an item of fascination for the hip and trendy, ever enchanted by all things proletariat. Thus the transgressive becomes normalized.

VI —— 005

What's the best way to offer someone a breath freshener?

Think twice about pulling out that old pack languishing in your jeans pocket: thigh-temp candy isn't exactly the most appetizing. Instead, keep a pack of gum in your jacket pocket. Then unwrap it like cigarettes and extend the open pack.

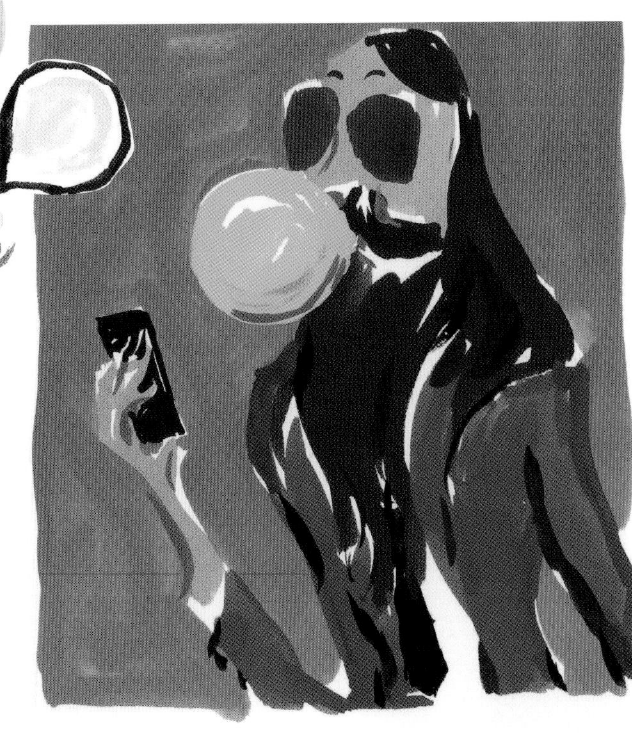

VI —— 006

WHAT'S WITH BLUE BLOODS AND LOUD COLORS?

It's the legacy of English fox hunting, with its bright red riding jackets. Put this together with a passion for fine arts and auction rooms on the one hand, and a preppy heritage—very colorful as well—on the other, and you get a loose interpretation of old-fashioned, larger-than-life cultural and social elitism.

VI —— 007

HOW CAN YOU BE A SUAVE METALHEAD?

Your collection of T-shirts featuring groups from this vast and pleasant musical genre is sufficiently full of tombstones and skulls. Your skinny jeans are black, your biker jacket shows just the right amount of wear, and you've just enough room on your body for another tattoo of the flames of hell. But rest assured, there are still a few avenues left to explore, starting with a denim or leather vest—kitsch and flamboyant.

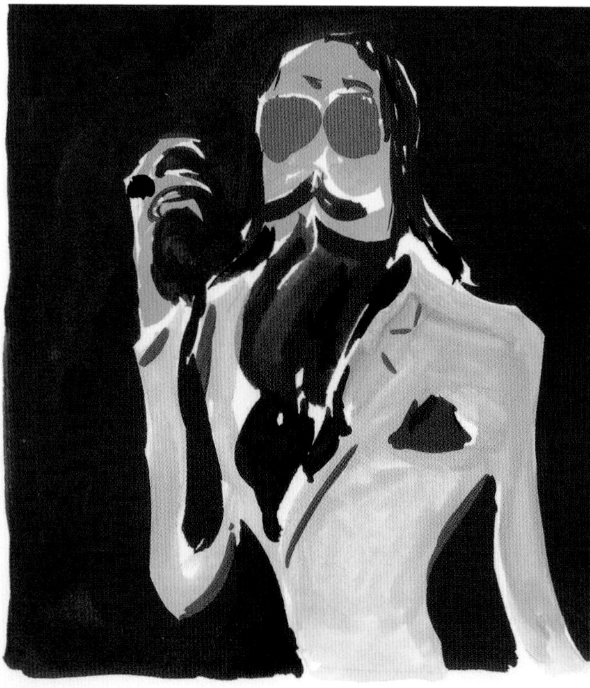

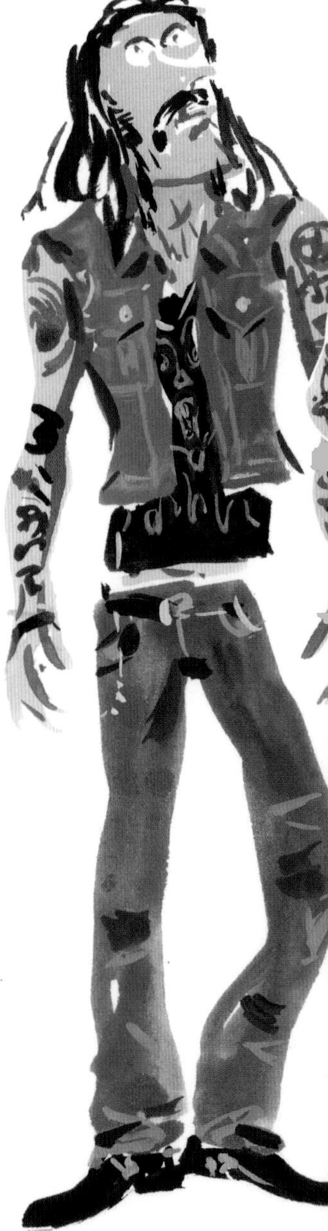

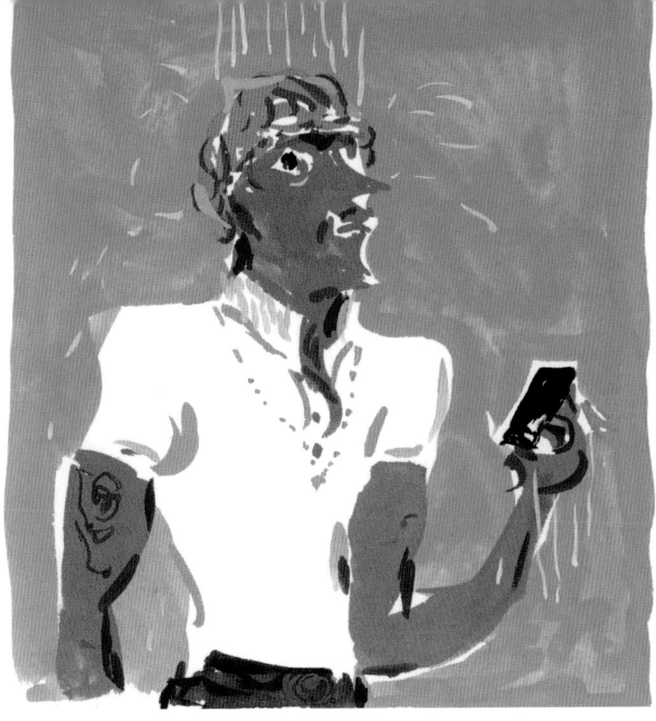

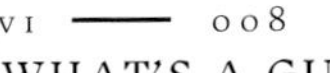

VI —— 008

WHAT'S A GUIDO?

A guido is the son of an aging party girl lost somewhere in a club on the Jersey shore and a dim-witted WWF fanatic with a Hulk Hogan thing. With such an auspicious start, he has learned that life comes down to reality TV shows, YouTube videos, and Ibiza club dance music compilation remixes. A guido does bodybuilding and tanning booths, uses hair gel by the quart, likes cheap tattoos (tribal or Chinese characters), Nascar races, boob jobs, customized jeans, curved sunglasses, and turned-up collars. Metrosexual, he takes everything literally and he really thinks he's the man. He poses for photos, smirking like the guy who just scored the winning touchdown in the Superbowl, and he's so self-absorbed he even takes selfies in the shower. At first glance he seems harmless, but he's hugely egotistical and totally in love with himself, enjoys getting on his friends' nerves, and thinks his fifteen minutes of fame should last forever. By extension, the term guido can be applied to anyone likely to make a display of his own idiocy. The fact remains that the next generation will see him differently: perhaps as amusing, since he embodies the idiocy of the times as few can. As everyone knows, it is in the garbage can of time that treasures are found and recycled.

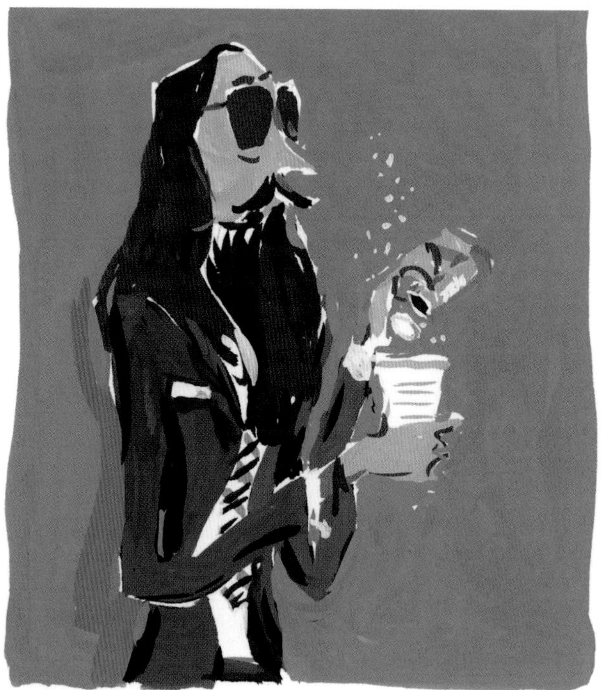

VI —— 009

WHAT'S THE BEST WAY TO DEAL WITH A HANGOVER?

Last night your coworkers took you to every college dive bar in town, and now that it's morning you look like five miles of bad road. Your first thought is to throw on your clothes from the night before. Huge mistake. You'll remain in the spirit of last night's revelries and will be caught whistling "Copacabana" to yourself. We suggest the opposite: stepping things up to tone things down, as it were. Dressed to the nines, you'll no longer look like a wino but a somewhat groggy charmer. Make sure you're so well dressed even the photocopier will blush. You'll be humming Miles Davis's soundtrack to Louis Malle's *Elevator to the Gallows* as you just about manage to stir your coffee. Your slight incoherence will be mistaken for wit. You are now the person you only dreamed of becoming. Congratulations.

VI —— 010

How should you dress when you're with people cooler than you?

Pressure land. Nothing could be better than a look that's out of step with fashion diktats. Why? Because to keep from following the herd, the king of cool is always one step ahead.

VI —— 011

SHOULD YOU RESIST THE BOWIE HYPE?

The disappearance of music greats such as Mötorhead's Lemmy Kilmister, David Bowie, Prince, Alan Vega, and Pierre Boulez has spurred a barrage of homages. In these moments of remembrance, seize the opportunity to show your discernment. Avoid discussions about Bowie's personality and don't wear T-shirts or whatnot with his effigy. Better still, keep quiet and go listen to some Leonard Cohen records.

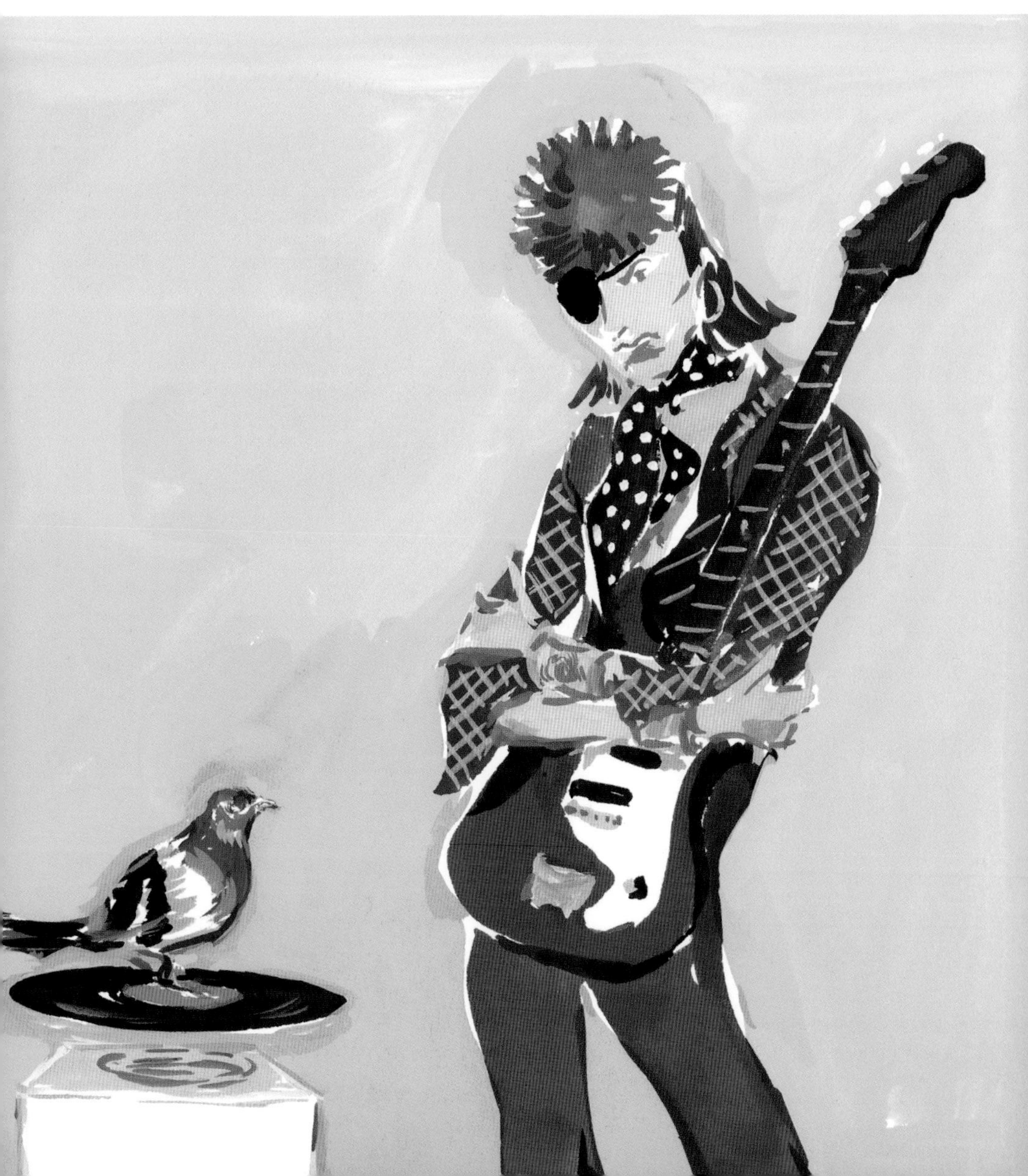

VI —— 012

HOW CAN YOU (MORE OR LESS) PULL OFF WEARING SUSPENDERS?

Two schools of thought come head to head over this thorny question: the old school against the older school, or rather, the punk versus the manual laborer. We're backing the hard-working little guys (model with buttons) over the faux anarchist pretty boys (clip-on style). We therefore recommend a button-down shirt, but forget the necktie and under no circumstances wear a T-shirt. For real proletariat style, ensure you roll your sleeves up the length of your forearm, stopping at the crook of your elbow. It goes without saying that your pants should feature buttons for attaching the suspenders.

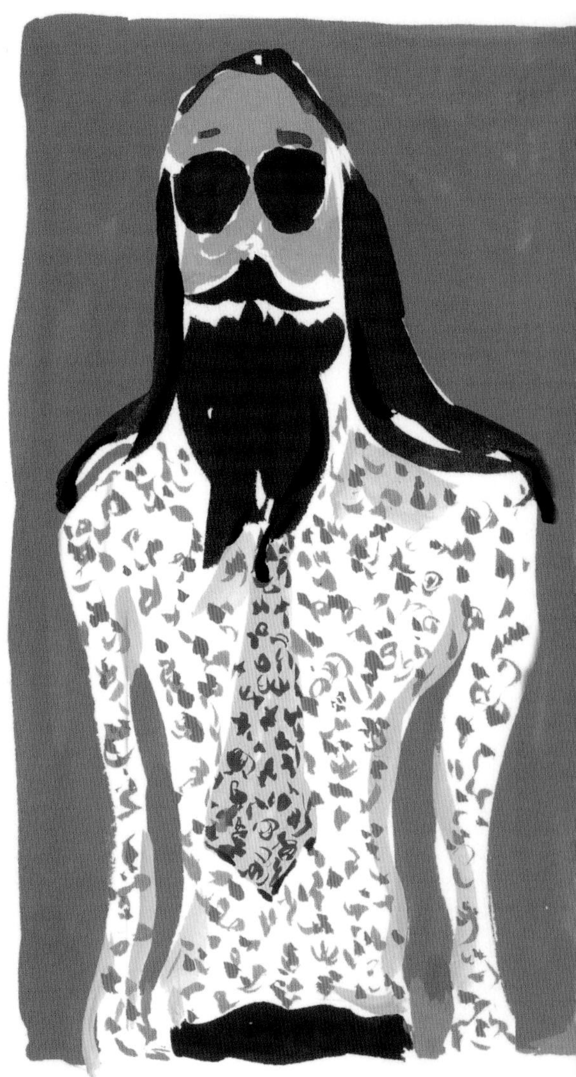

VI —— 013

SHOULD YOU GO FOR A FLORAL PRINT?

Naturally. Or, rather, it depends. I mean, our British friends like to express their poetic natures come rain or shine. That's why they print little flowers on their shirts. Liberty shirts are, however, a summer option not to be undertaken lightly. Tradition dictates that the print be worn with a linen suit, but you run the risk of looking like an aging dandy. We recommend wearing it with jeans on the weekend, just unkempt enough for a new romantic vibe. This picnic spirit *à la* open house at the University of Manchester's Humanities department should see you through, whatever the weather.

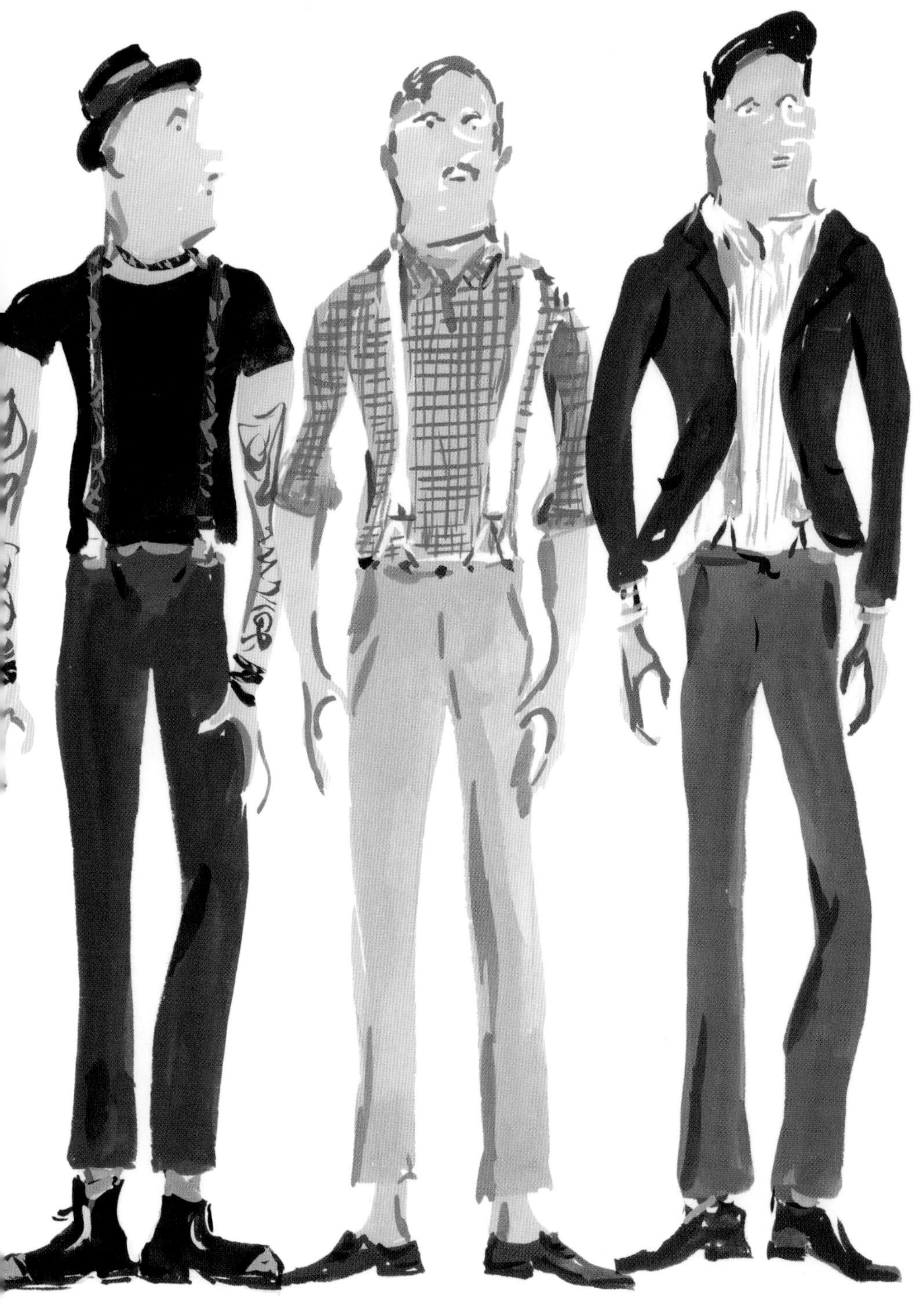

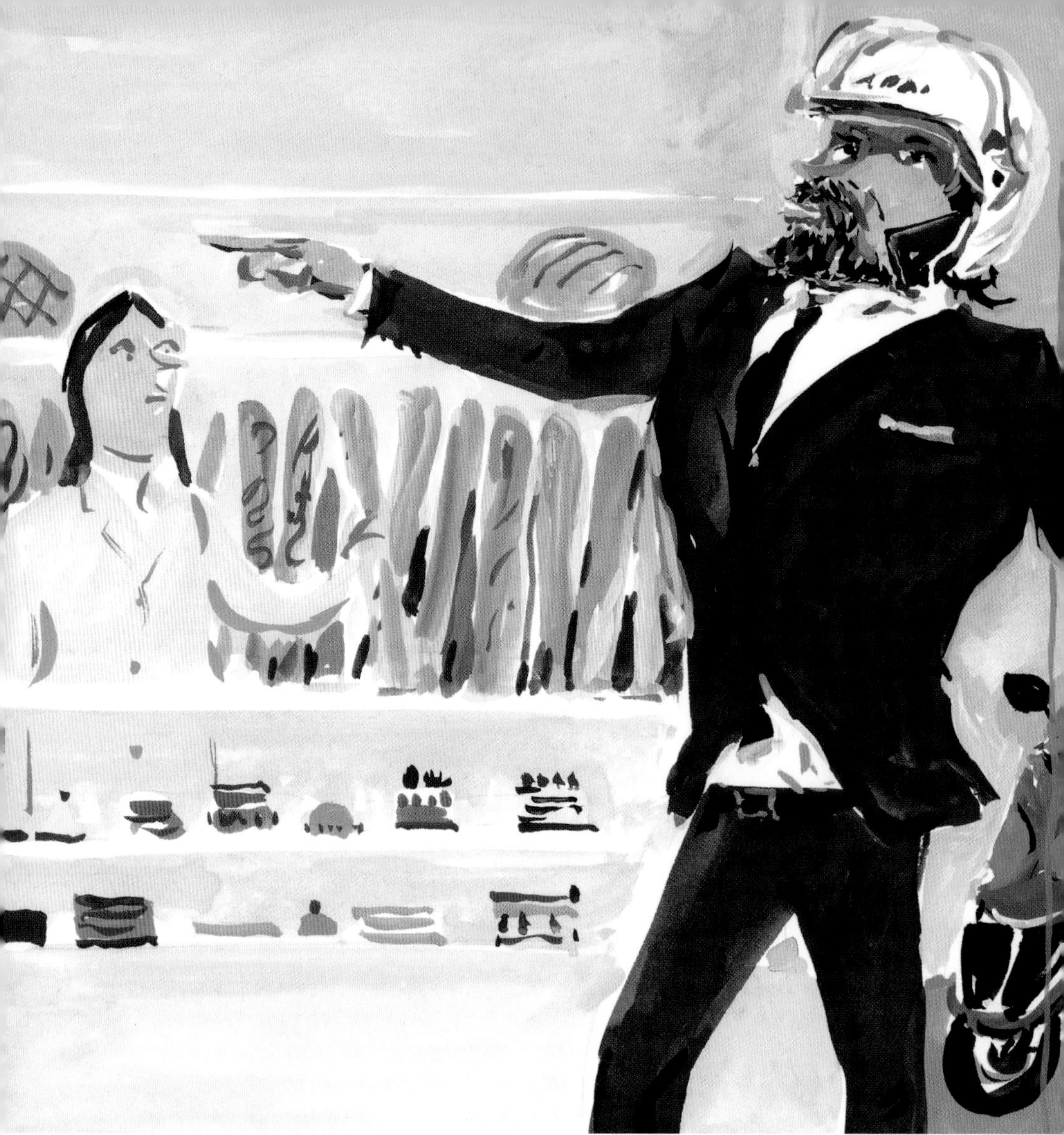

VI —— 014

CAN YOU KEEP YOUR HELMET ON AT THE BAKERY?

Keeping your helmet on in a public place is a sign of disdain. He who sees himself as an exemplary gentleman of the road should learn to blend in more with the masses. Your helmet, politely held in your hand, gives you a certain charm, all the better for getting service when you're ordering your almond croissants and *pains au chocolat.* Only professional bikers—such as pizza deliverymen and human-organ couriers—or knights may keep their headgear on when entering a public place. They just need to lift their visor.

VI —— 015

WHERE DOES THE CHINSTRAP BEARD COME FROM?

It originated as a form of religious traditionalism (the beard), toned down by the removal of the mustache. Whether spiritual or seductive, it's hot.

VI —— 016

IS IT OK TO WEAR A RUSSIAN HAT IN AN ELEVATOR?

Let's consider this carefully: when you wear a Russian fur cap—an *ushanka*—you look like a schmuck. Thus we strongly advise you to take the stairs. If you're wearing a more distinguished accessory on your head, it is best to take it off in the presence of ladies. This may be third-rate gallantry, an outdated reflex from days gone by, but it shows you're not a jerk. If you are not waiting for the elevator alone, let the women enter first, then keep your hat on your head. Otherwise, depending on its size, it can take up room for nothing (same goes for backpacks). On the other hand, if you are alone in the elevator, wear whatever the hell you want, no matter how ridiculous. It's nobody's business but yours.

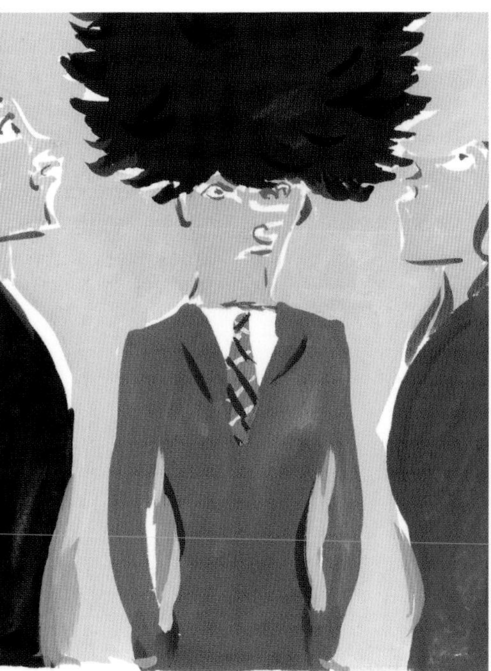

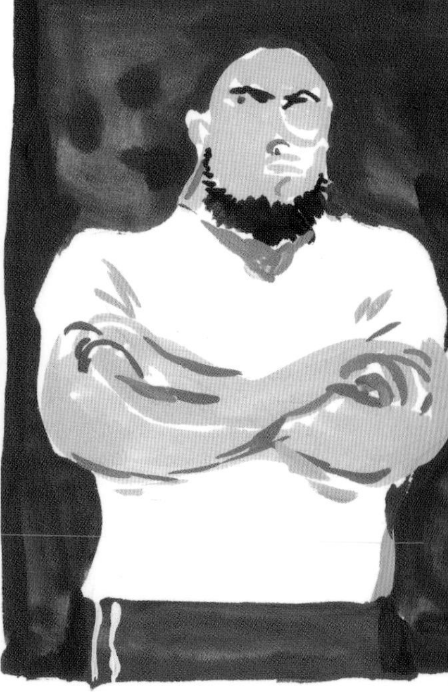

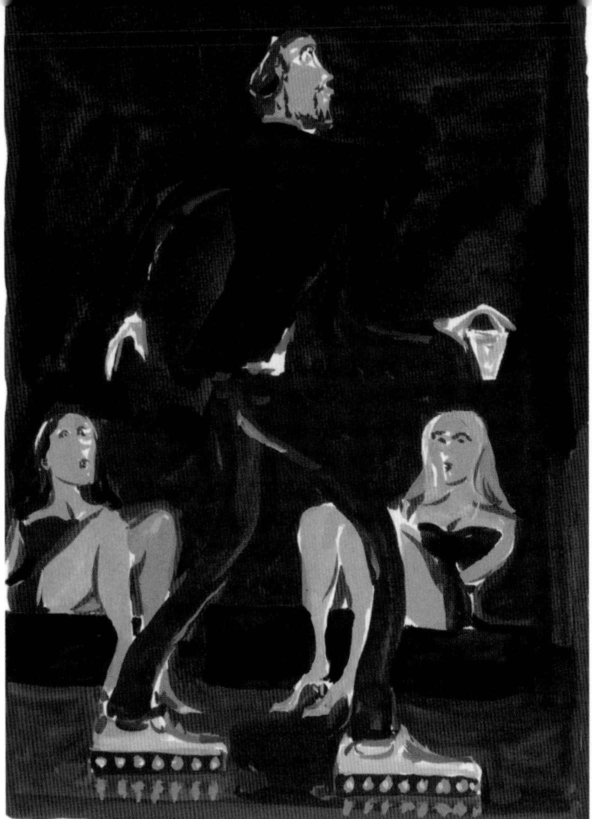

VI —— 017

WHAT'S THE VERDICT ON SNEAKERS WITH FLASHING SOLES?

In the name of research, we once called in mature French actor Jean Rochefort—the ultimate in suave—to test out a hoverboard. He came to our aid once again to help us judge those sneakers with LED soles that light up as you walk. So there we were with Jean, imagining ourselves in *Avatar*'s magic forest or on the dance floor at the Gotha Club during the Cannes film festival, in keeping with the fantasy world conjured up by these shoes. Although we have refrained from rushing out to buy a pair, our world lights up every time we come across them.

VI —— 018

ARE PRE-TIED BOW TIES ACCEPTABLE?

The quest for simplicity naturally spurs you to say yes, but don't lose sight of the fact that we are talking about style here. Since you can now read our minds, you understand perfectly that wearing a bow tie requires some effort, and it is worn with all its imperfections. It's a little like your shoelace knot: after a few unsuccessful attempts, you will soon become a gentleman who is every bit as autonomous as he is demanding.

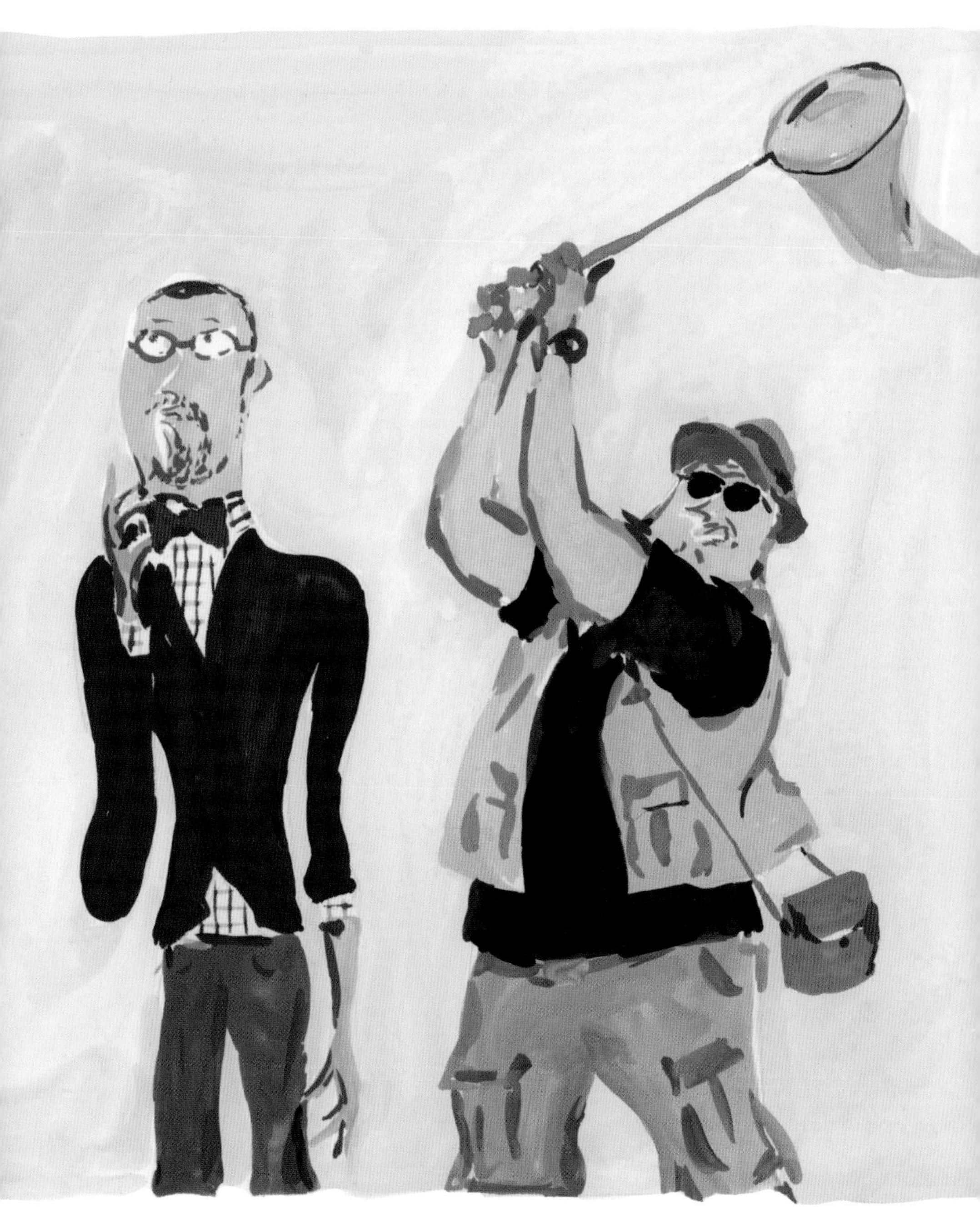

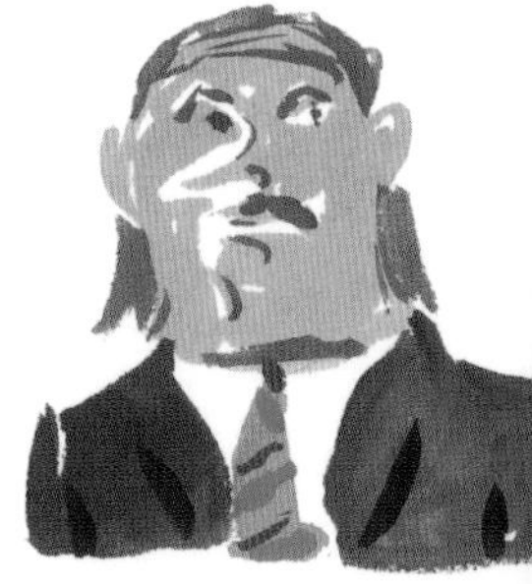

VI —— 019

WHY CUT OFF YOUR SWEATSHIRT AT THE ELBOWS?

Steve McQueen (5 ft. 8 in. / 1.77 m), Sylvester Stallone (5 ft. 8 in. / 1.77 m), Eddy Murphy (5 ft. 7½ in. / 1.75 m), Kanye West (5 ft. 7 in. / 1.73 m): the world's greatest style icons have always looked taller thanks to this trick, which is now yours to try.

VI —— 020

WHICH HAIR ISSUES ARE MUCH ADO ABOUT NOTHING?

1. The comb-over. Valery Giscard d'Estaing, Prince Charles, Joe Biden, Abdelaziz Bouteflika: all have chosen to deal with reality by hiding the top of their head rather than holding their head in their hands. Be a big wig like them. 2. Red hair. Though tormented spirits Richard D. James (alias Aphex Twin, the British genius of electro) and Guns n' Roses singer Axl Rose didn't always help matters, redheads are finally witnessing a return to favor. 3. Curls. Sorry, but perfectly smooth hair is not the be-all and end-all to be adopted by the entire planet. We need a little zaniness! Let your curls be. Don't try to tame them by parting your hair on the side. 4. Baldness. We celebrate its poetry and, on occasion, we cover it with a hat that highlights its existence. A huge shout out to *Breaking Bad*'s Bryan Cranston, who got the tip from Kojak.

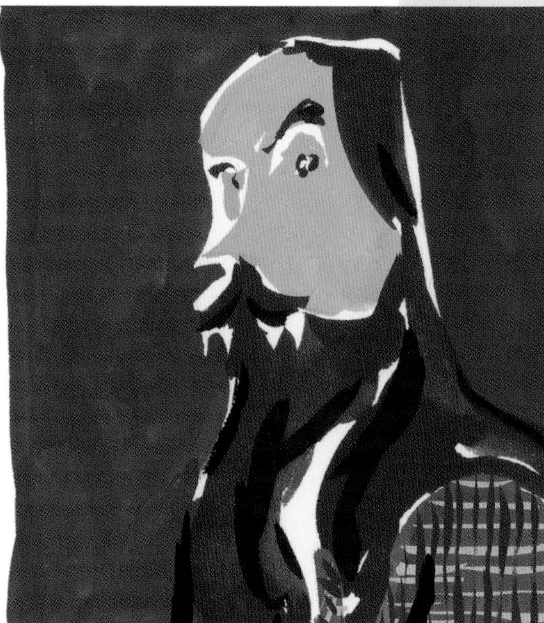

VI —— 021

Should you "werk it" with your eyebrows?

My goodness. Squinting is good, but knowing how to use the muscle power of your eyebrow is a thousand times better. Show your disapproval and your surprise, or give someone a killer look with the help of this trick, used by all the world's greatest gentlemen.

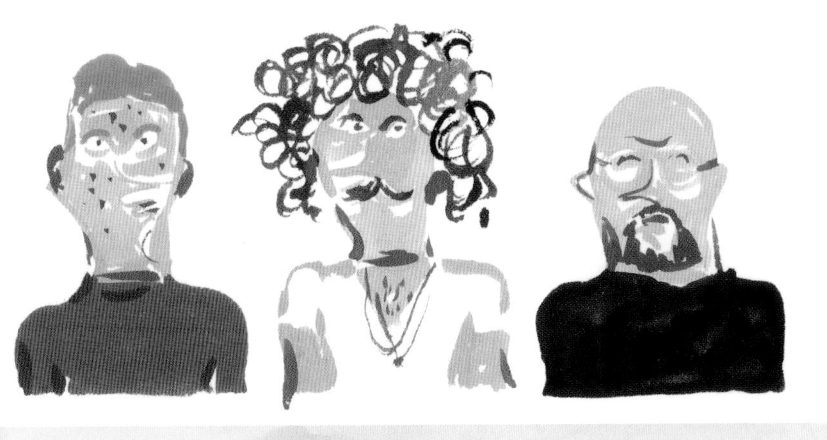

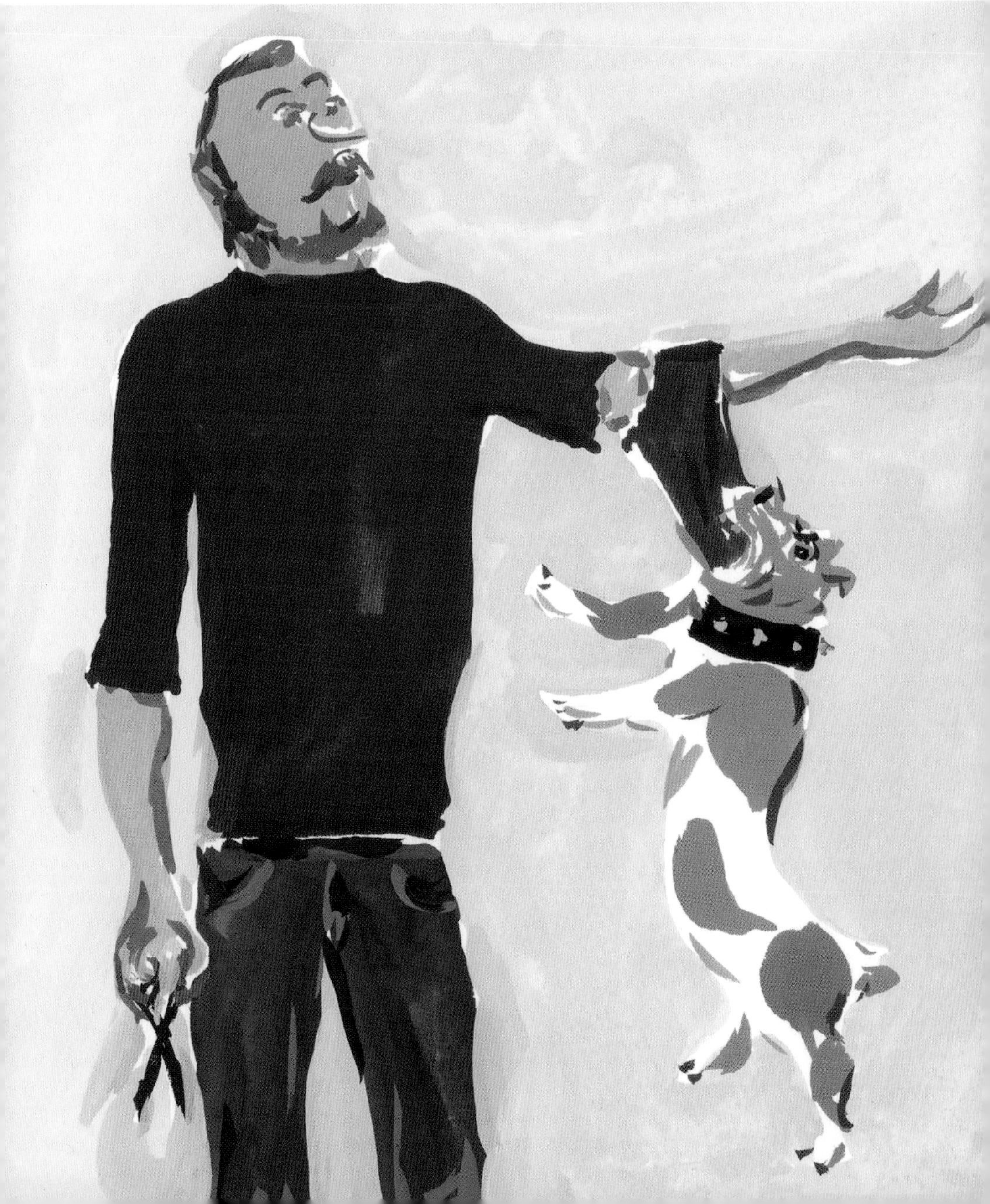

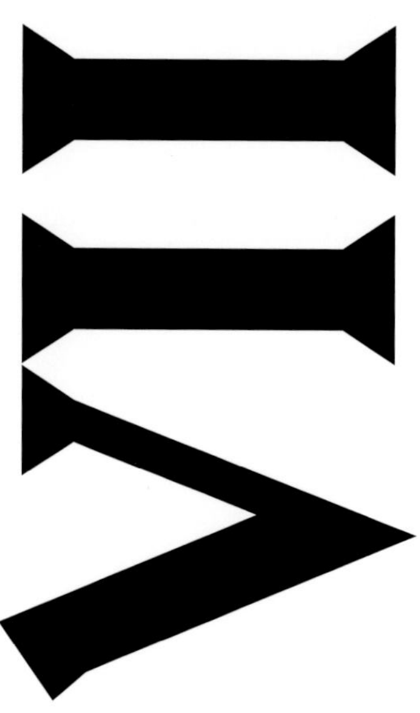

PLAY UP YOUR

VII —— 001 › VII —— 023

How does a turtleneck enhance virility? • How can you score points in an open-plan office? • Is it ok to smile with only one side of your mouth, à la Peter Sellers? • What should you wear to a funeral? • How can you grab the waiter's (and only the waiter's) attention? • Which suave James Bond villain has the best secret weapon to steal? • Should you succumb to a smartwatch? • What is a bigotelle? • On vacation, can you tie your shirttails at the waist? • How can you get "Britítude"? • Is the Pacific seahorse the last of the great romantics? • How should you behave when the buffet opens? • How can you tell the difference between a good hunter

PANACHE

and a bad one? • At work, why would you fake a phone call? • In the car, is it ok for the backseat passenger seated in the middle to talk into the driver's ear? • Can you smoke a cigarette while talking on the phone? • What do Mike Hammer, Alain Delon, and Marcello Mastroianni have in common? • Which swimming stroke is the most elegant? • What are the essentials of the ultimate in suave style? • How can you avoid slipping when you're wearing new shoes? • How can you look like a biker without the ride? • Should you speak a foreign language with the best possible accent? • What should you wear when the weather sizzles?

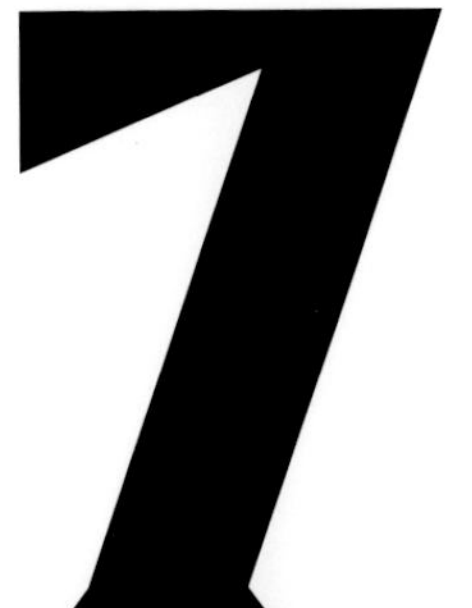

CHAPTER SEVEN

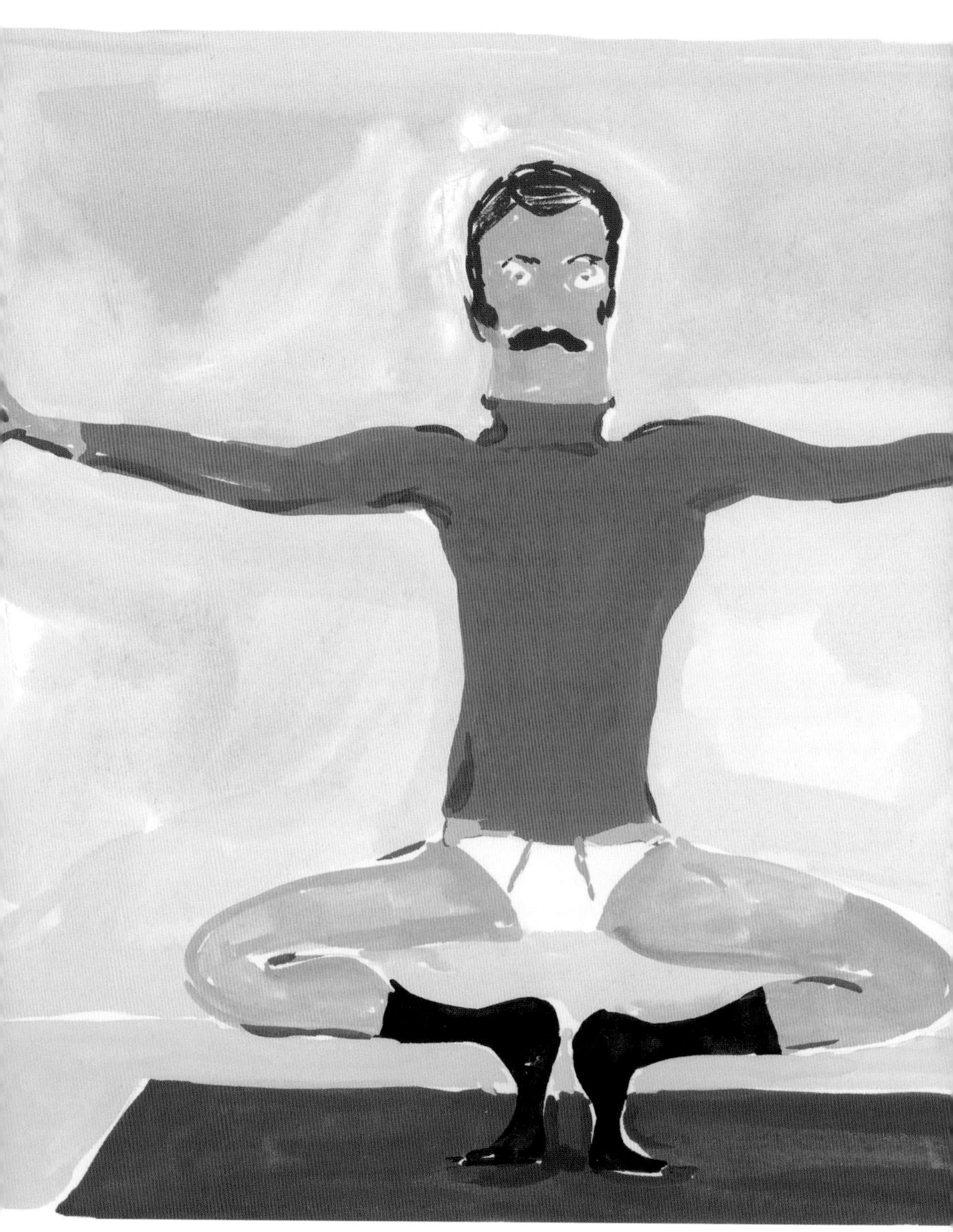

PLAY UP YOUR PANACHE

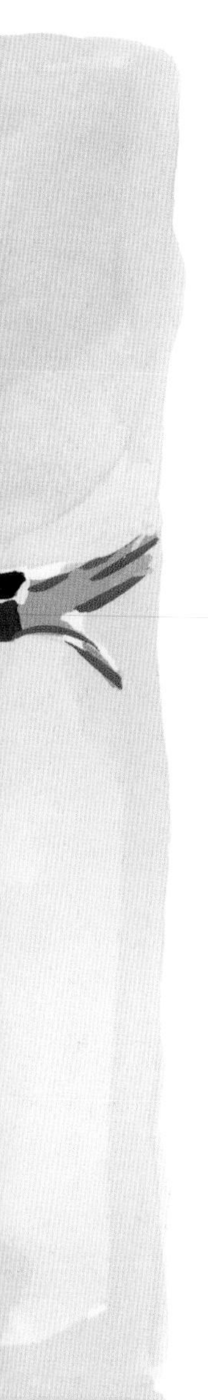

VII —— 001

HOW DOES A TURTLENECK ENHANCE VIRILITY?

Navy blue for old sea dogs; white Shetland wool for prep school boys; pure black for existentialists and intellectuals; and bright colors for provocateurs: the turtleneck is a sporty garment that became a utopian futurist symbol in the late 1960s. Forget the myth that it adds a few pounds: its tight fit flatters a beefy athletic build, bringing out the alpha male that lies somewhere within you. Further interpretations include the Freudian association of the neck with the foreskin, and experts in body language have identified the nape as the symbolic seat of self-confidence. Taken together, all evidence points toward the verdict that the turtleneck exudes virility. This is why the proper way to wear one—preferably under a fitted jacket with wide lapels, or a leather jacket for thicker versions—is a matter of either dispute or admiration.

VII —— 002

HOW CAN YOU SCORE POINTS IN AN OPEN-PLAN OFFICE?

1. Around each group, be warm and generous with your sense of humor. Though you are very well brought up and mostly sensitive to those around you, you realize you can be a bit much at times. 2. Retreat as necessary, lower your ringtone to its lowest setting, make your calls at a distance from others, modulate your voice to suit the size of your audience, and take a break every ninety minutes to rid yourself of any badly channeled energy before it backfires on you.

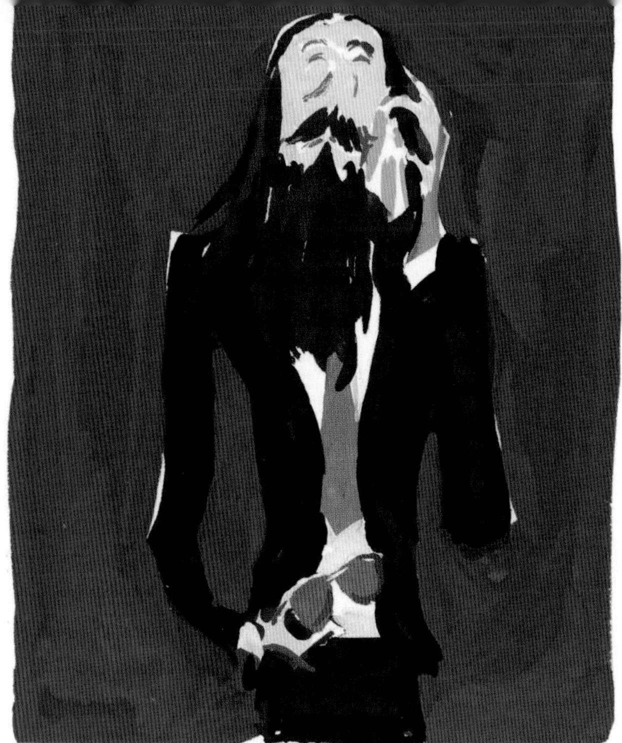

VII — 003

IS IT OK TO SMILE WITH ONLY ONE SIDE OF YOUR MOUTH, *À LA* PETER SELLERS?

No, unfortunately. No one will get it. You'll look as though your face is paralyzed. Save it for another time. To look great in a photo, smile as naturally as possible. Small, pinched mouths should be stretched to a maximum. Large or big-lipped mouths can be overly expressive and should be made more discreet. A slight lift of the zygomaticus major muscle is all it takes. P.S.: If you persist in goofing around and sporting a half-smile, remember to raise the opposite eyebrow at least.

VII — 004

What should you wear to a funeral?

In a black suit, black tie, and white shirt, you'll be taken for funeral parlor staff. Wear dark clothing, but not your finest attire, as the circumstances don't call for it. It goes without saying that a pale, cold-colored tie will cheer up the gloomy ceremony to which you have been invited.

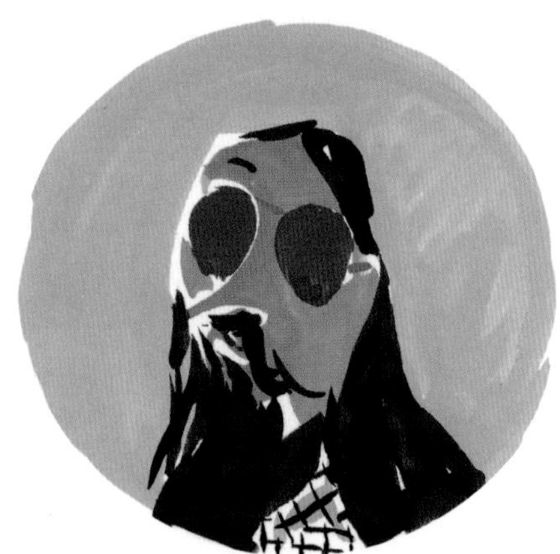

VII —— 005

HOW CAN YOU GRAB THE WAITER'S (AND ONLY THE WAITER'S) ATTENTION?

You want to ask for a pitcher of water or the check, but the damn waiter doesn't see you. Calm down, doggone it! To gesture for attention, keep your raised hand within your field of vision, about twenty inches from your face, your thumb no higher than your forehead. Apart from your slightly stretched index, the fingers are relaxed, your wrist extended—a cross between Michelangelo's *The Creation of Adam* and Jesus Christ.

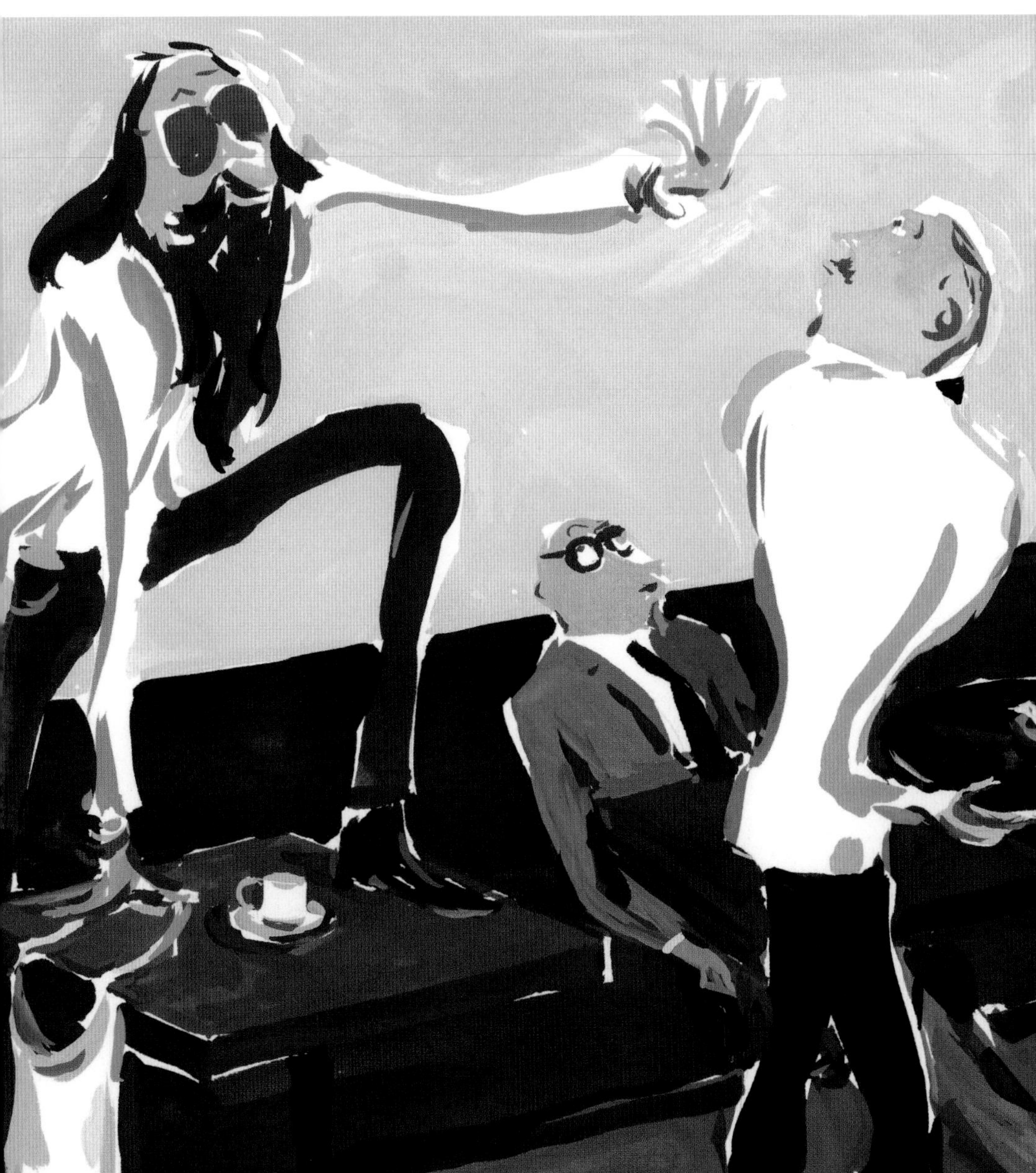

VII —— 006

WHICH SUAVE *JAMES BOND* VILLAIN HAS THE BEST SECRET WEAPON TO STEAL?

The coolest gang in the whole 007 series appears in *Live and Let Die* (1973), where Roger Moore comes head to head with veritable fashion warriors. Tee Hee has a metal arm. Another character is the voodoo incarnation of Baron Samedi (or else a mortal in his guise). All the villains sport suits with wide lapels and brightly colored silk ties (our favorites feature bold patterns that look like shells or crosses). This is not a look for the faint-hearted.

VII —— 007

SHOULD YOU SUCCUMB TO A SMARTWATCH?

The Internet of Things—the IoT—is changing our way of life. Eventually, the information gathered by smartwatches and smart T-shirts will be used to notify the emergency services of a problem, or by insurance agents to renegotiate our medical expenses. Until then, don't allow your wrist to pass judgment on your lifestyle. If you can't do without one, we suggest a watch model with hands for a more universal notion of the passage of time.

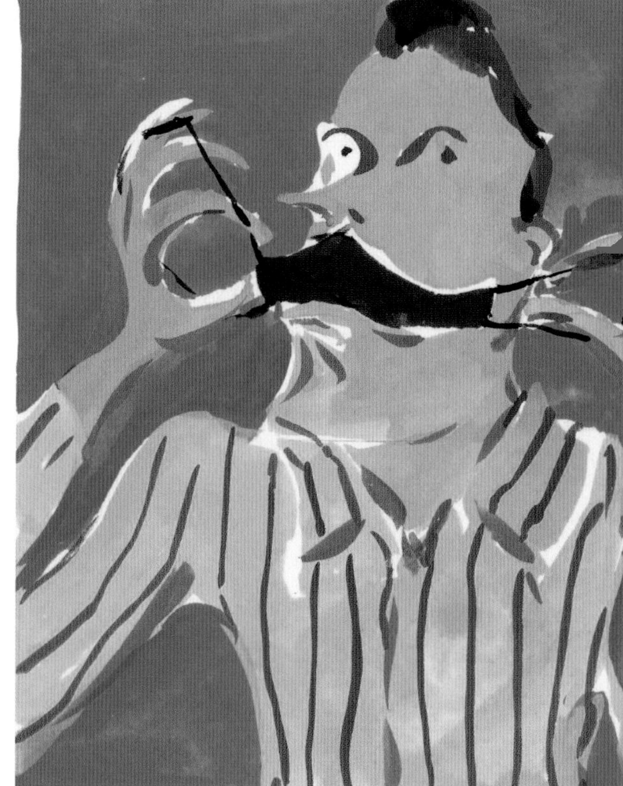

VII —— 008

What is a *bigotelle*?

It's a sort of sleeping cap for a mustache. After brushing your facial hair, you cover it overnight with a piece of cloth or leather that is held in place with straps that hook over your ears. In the same spirit, you can also wear a hairnet to keep your part straight.

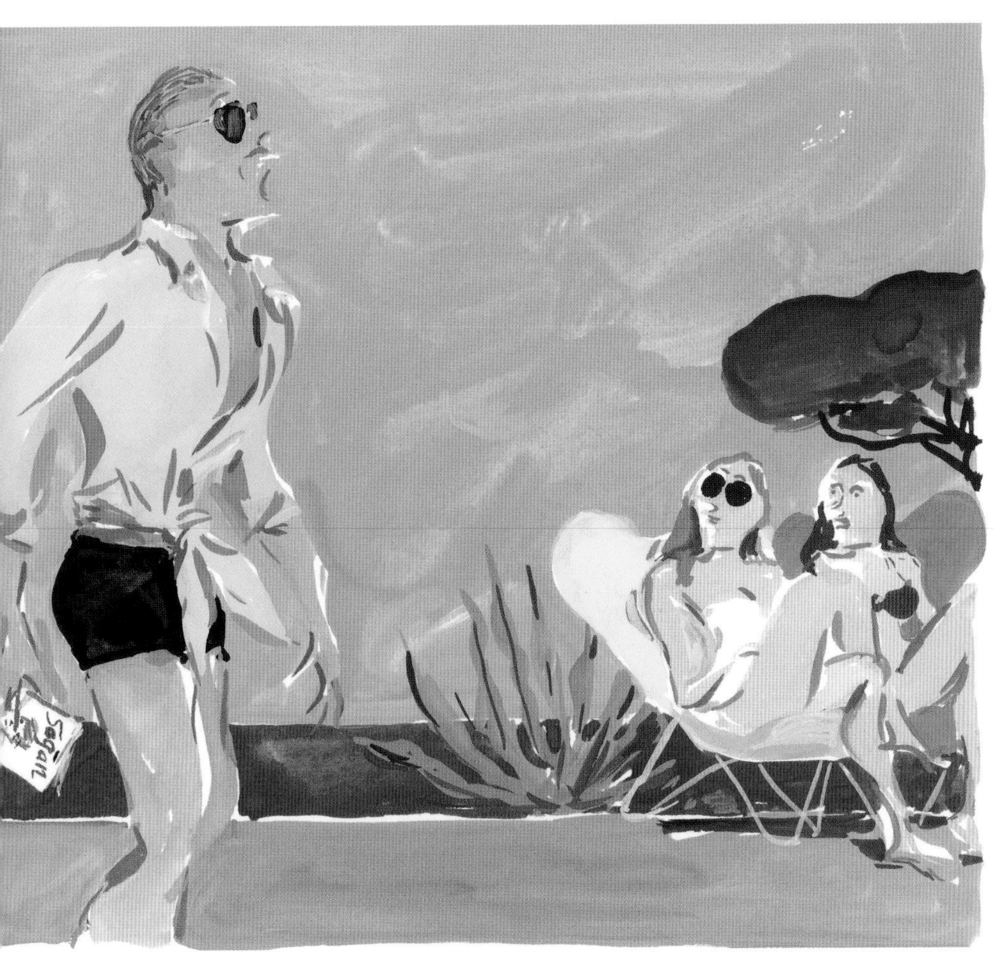

VII —— 009

ON VACATION, CAN YOU TIE YOUR SHIRTTAILS AT THE WAIST?

Only if you are a twentieth-century playboy—especially the kind seen in movies recounting their extraordinary adventures on the French Riviera. Take David Niven, for example, in Otto Preminger's *Bonjour Tristesse* (1958). The charm he exerts over Jean Seberg is undeniable. Unfortunately, it's highly unlikely that, in the height of summer, the same will be true of you. So keep your shirt—in lightweight fabric, of course—sensibly on your back. If necessary, open it slightly to reveal your chest, whether hairy, smooth, tanned, or pale.

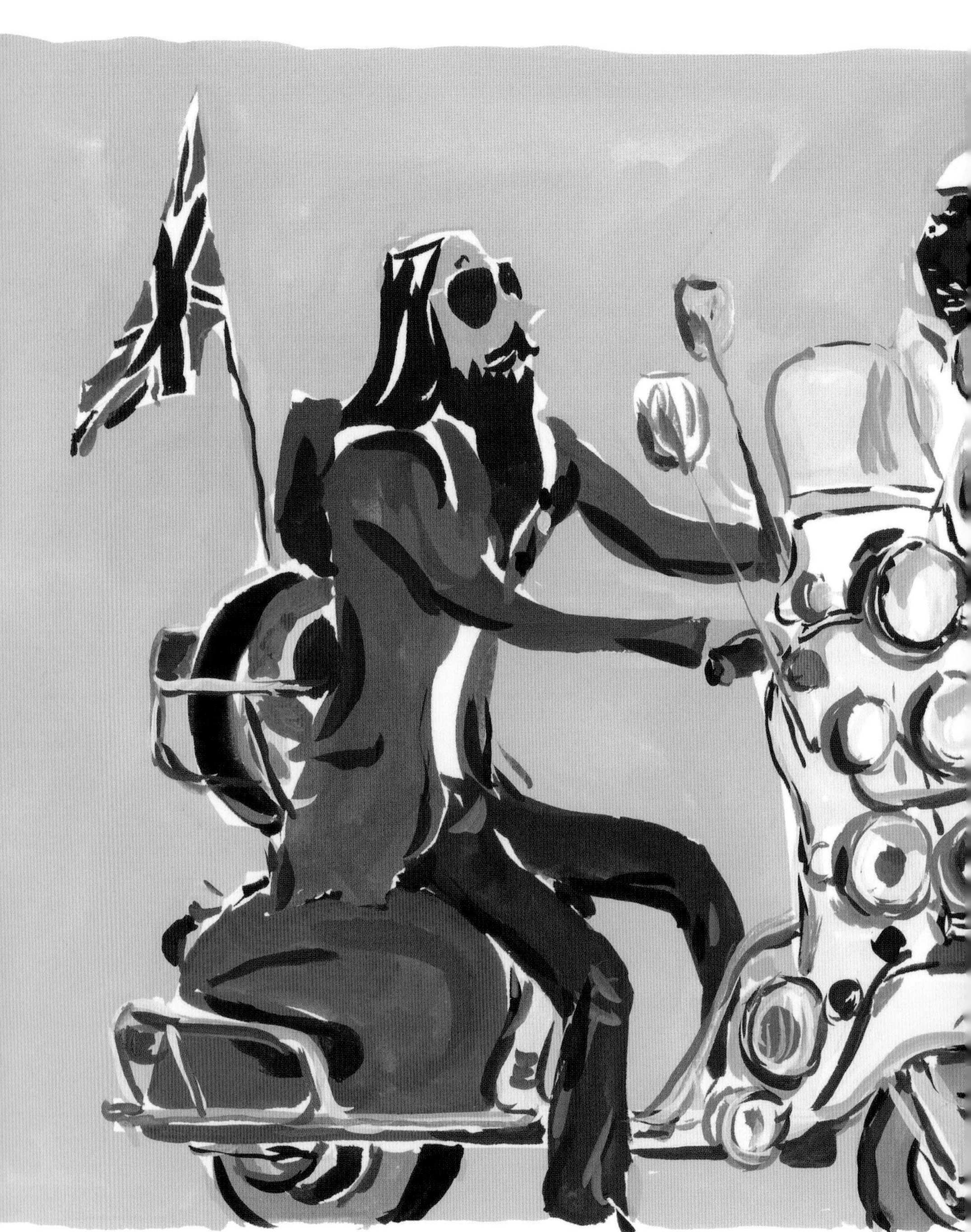

PLAY UP YOUR PANACHE

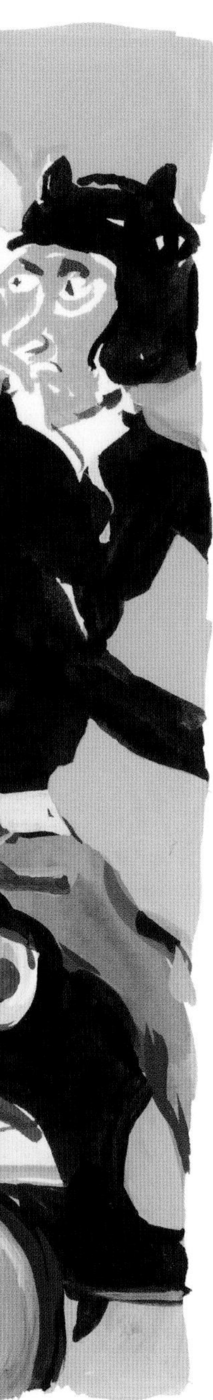

VII — 010

HOW CAN YOU GET "BRITITUDE"?

Working-class cockiness and aristocratic composure divide Her Majesty's subjects. Option 1: on a motor scooter in a fitted suit, you're a blue-collar gentleman—a lad, a mod, a diamond geezer. With open disdain, stare straight into people's eyes, unblinking. Hold your cigarette between your thumb and index finger. Don't bark; let things go awry on their own. Bare your teeth; very few people actually want to fight. Option 2: holding your head high, give the person you are speaking to a sideways glance. Hold your cigarette between your index and middle fingers, drawing on it slowly and affectedly. Always articulate, with an even tone of voice. Coolly send adversaries to hell. Show no sign of emotion. In high circles, scandal doesn't tarnish: it kills.

VII — 011

IS THE PACIFIC SEAHORSE THE LAST OF THE GREAT ROMANTICS?

The direct descendant of a line as old as the formation of Mount Everest (some fifty million years), the seahorse is a member of the same family as the highly appreciated pipefish. The male Pacific seahorse is distinguished by its haughty demeanor and old-fashioned disdain. Its extremely fine skin, stretched over a frail skeleton, is both ghoulish and sublime. It is a lazy and discreet creature by nature, with a coolness that hides just how much of a rascal it is. Proof of this lies in the elaborateness of its courtship dance, which is choreographed like a Bolshoi ballet. Narcissistic, it holds the masculine ideal in such high esteem that it even carries the eggs and gives birth to its offspring. The rest of the time, it sleeps in the coral reefs, moored to algae masses by its prehensile tail and sucking up the micro shrimp on offer.

VII — 012

HOW SHOULD YOU BEHAVE WHEN THE BUFFET OPENS?

Either you are the instigator, in which case you should smilingly invite everyone to join the line; or you wait—without a plastic plate in hand or showing any irritation—for a good part of the crowd to have served themselves before you partake yourself. You are surrounded by people who think with their stomach, and that's fine. By definition, a gentleman is a role model. He is the mirror, reflecting the world as it should be—ruled by the heart, not the stomach.

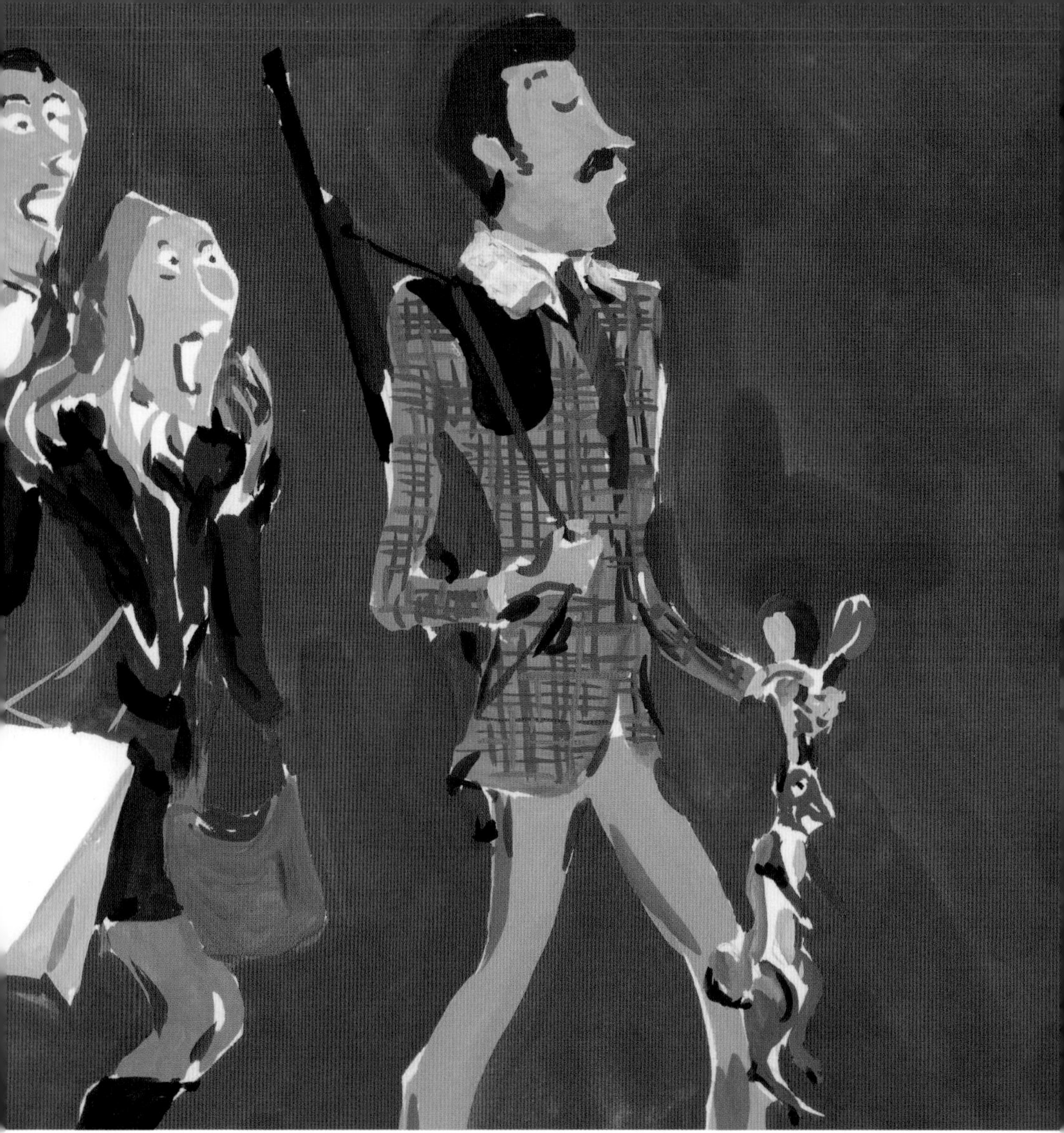

VII —— 013

HOW CAN YOU TELL THE DIFFERENCE BETWEEN A GOOD HUNTER AND A BAD ONE?

You can spot a real hunter by the yoke stitched to the shoulder of his jacket, where the butt of the rifle can rest without sliding off. He is then free to miss his target without shooting off his partner's toe. Today this piece, often in leather or suede, is but a relic of a violent past. It is now primarily a joining technique for garments (to attach the back to the front and sleeves), guaranteeing greater ease of movement (when jostling with your neighboring hunter for example). Note that it is entirely possible to be taken for a hunter in the city. Or taken for prey. It's up to you.

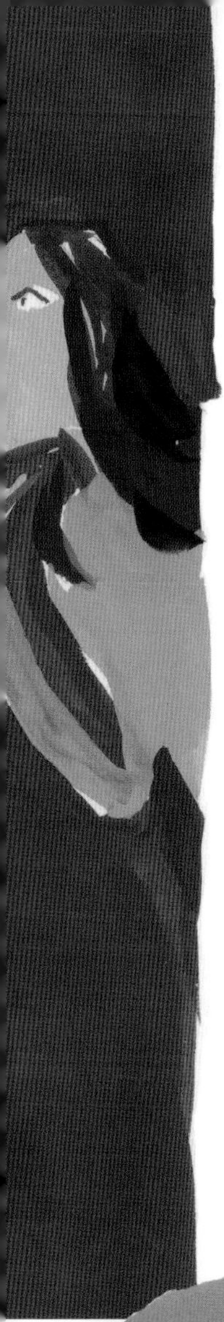

VII —— 014

AT WORK, WHY WOULD YOU FAKE A PHONE CALL?

When you need to heed the call of nature while at the office, you need to have a good alibi ready. Seated with your head down, unlock your cell phone. Then stand up and head toward the nearest hallway, pretending to flick through your numbers in search of that golden contact in your list. In one natural movement, stick your mobile solution to your ear; you should place the other hand in your pocket. If you run into colleagues on the way to your destination, look like you are waiting for the other person to pick up or listening intently to a voice-mail message. The rest is up to you. Don't get caught doing the same thing when you come back, or your secret will be out and you'll be the butt of jokes.

VII —— 015

IN THE CAR, IS IT OK FOR THE BACKSEAT PASSENGER SEATED IN THE MIDDLE TO TALK INTO THE DRIVER'S EAR?

Apart from the fact that, without his seatbelt, this person risks shooting through the windshield like a cannonball, we believe this seat should be kept for the passenger who knows best how to prevent the driver from nodding off.

VII —— 016

CAN YOU SMOKE A CIGARETTE WHILE TALKING ON THE PHONE?

While smoking may work in your favor when playing out your film noir fantasies, it will often diminish your charm over the telephone, punctuating your conversation with inhaling and exhaling sounds. We therefore formally declare a ban on cigarette-smoking on the phone—in fact, in any situation in which the other party is deprived of the view of this smoky spectacle emerging from your mouth.

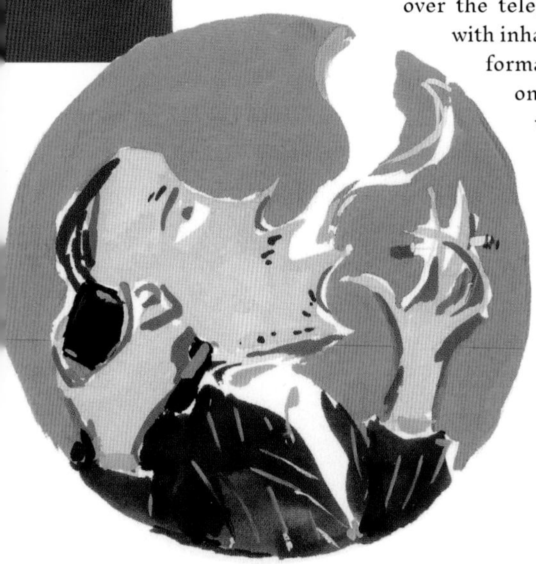

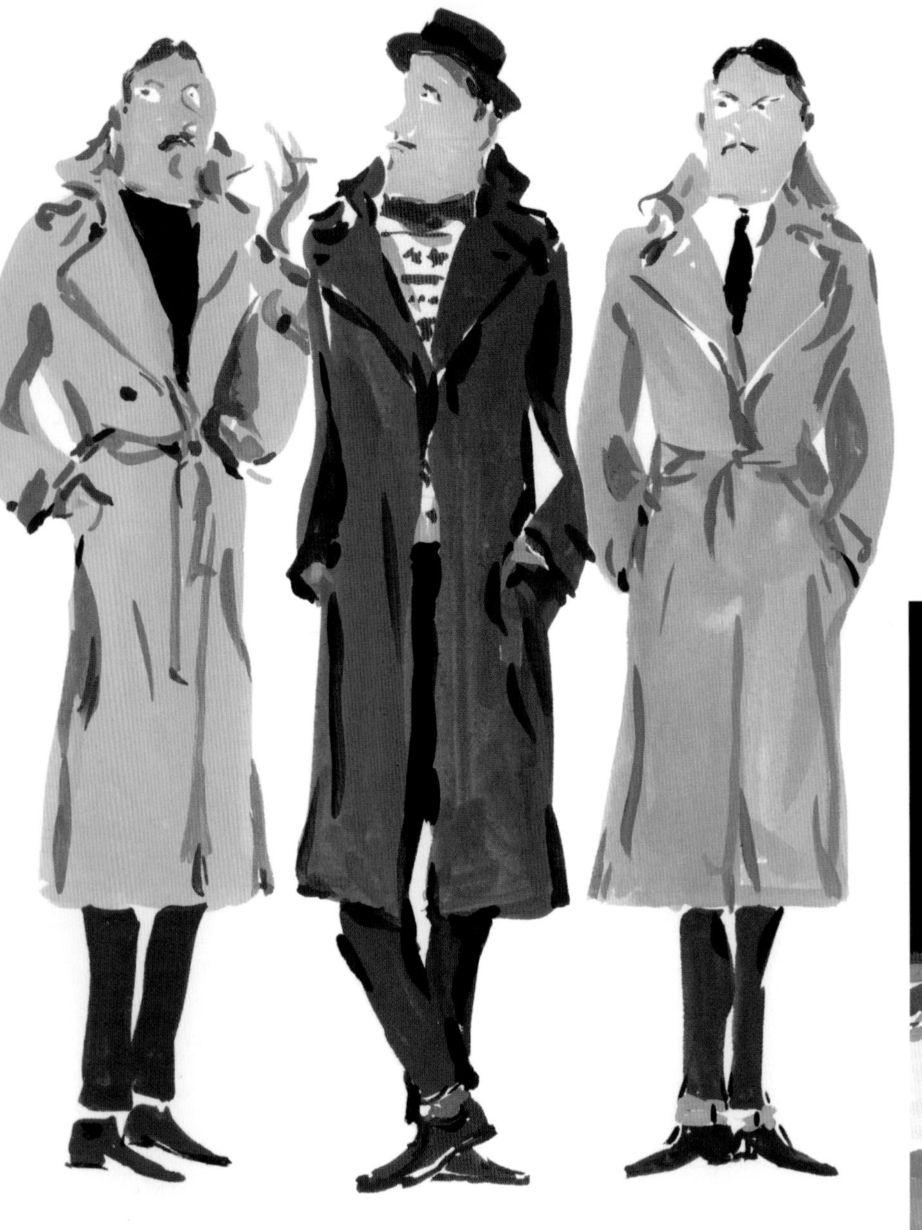

VII —— 017

WHAT DO MIKE HAMMER, ALAIN DELON, AND MARCELLO MASTROIANNI HAVE IN COMMON?

All three have a distinctive way of turning up the collar on their raincoat, whether trench or mackintosh. Unlike the crude style of the tall, dark, well-heeled guy who'd like to think he's Humphrey Bogart but doesn't even measure up to Hugh Laurie's ankle, this is an approach that we call the "French *GQ* style." It has no clear instructions. The best we can say is, turn up your collar after folding it along the neckline.

VII —— 018

WHICH SWIMMING STROKE IS THE MOST ELEGANT?

The one that takes you as far as the buoys. If you are of a modest constitution, give in to the joys of the sidestroke. And whatever category you are in, remember to swim parallel to the beach. There are two reasons for this: it keeps you from drowning at sea and it offers onlookers a veritable cinematographic panorama. If you're a stalwart front-crawl fan, remember that you must keep your head in the water and alternate breathing on the left and right sides, otherwise you're unworthy of putting on a show. Finally, the first person who pretends to do the butterfly will eat a fistful of sand.

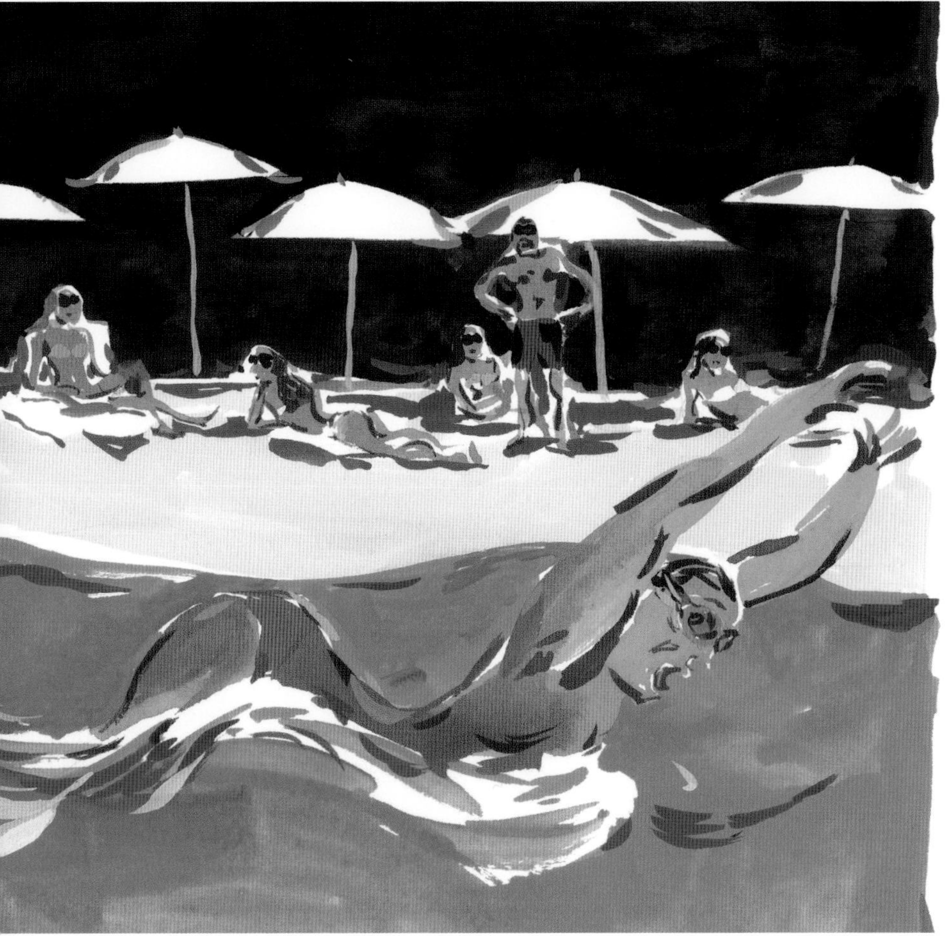

VII —— 019

WHAT ARE THE ESSENTIALS OF THE ULTIMATE IN SUAVE STYLE?

The sartorial style of the French writer and gentleman-charmer Jean d'Ormesson—the epitome of suave—has been the same since the invention of television. It comprises: 1. A "Lanvin blue" end-to-end shirt from Hilditch & Key (Jermyn Street, London) or Carven (France), which matches the color of his eyes. 2. A black silk or black wool necktie with a square end (Uniqlo has offered square-end ties, which are perfect imitations of his, at a fraction of the cost). 3. Four two-button jackets: in gray flannel, gray coarse wool, blue cashmere, and beige gabardine, for summer. "Materials that have a soul, for this connoisseur," explains his tailor. 4. A classic pair of trousers, with two pleats and cuffs, and matching jacket. 5. A pocket square. 6. Blue socks (in Italy, they say black is for chauffeurs): lisle in summer, wool in winter. To the knee, of course. 7. A pair of bespoke black Berluti shoes, even though, lately, Mr. d'Ormesson has grown a bit tired of them. Otherwise, the Perrier model—a six-hole classic derby from John Lobb. Again, and as ever, bespoke. 8. The French Legion of Honor medal (today practically anybody can get one). 9. An impeccable haircut. 10. Bedroom eyes. 11. Skillful rhetoric. 12. An extra-white smile. Rid yourself of all hang-ups—that would look ridiculous. Because Jean also wears jeans. Slim fit, of course! Would you kindly note that he has never given his attire the slightest twist. It is revolutionary in its excellence and its consistency.

VII —— 020

HOW CAN YOU AVOID SLIPPING WHEN YOU'RE WEARING NEW SHOES?

You should place rubber anti-slip soles on your shoes, but we recommend wearing in the leather of the sole a little, ahead of time, by rubbing your foot on asphalt or gravel. Enjoy a quiet moment alone to complete this task, because no one wants to be seen dragging their feet. Otherwise, with the tip of a pair of scissors, lightly score the sole where it touches the ground, as though scoring the fat on a duck breast. Bear in mind, however, that anti-slip soles can seriously harm your attempts at sliding around on the dance floor when you really want to cut loose.

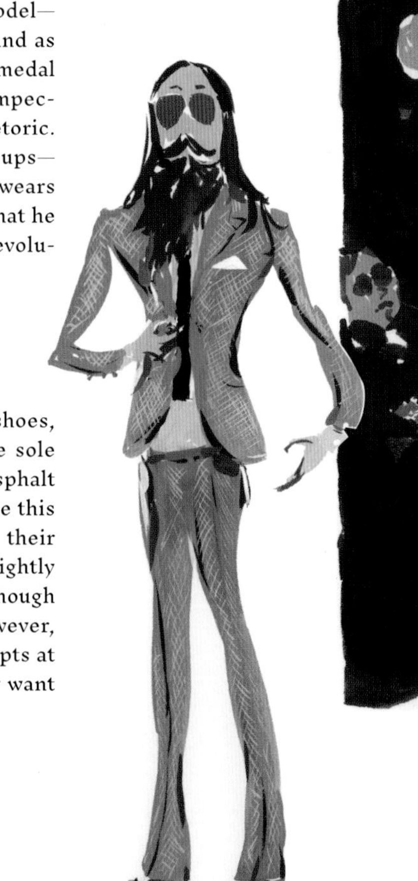

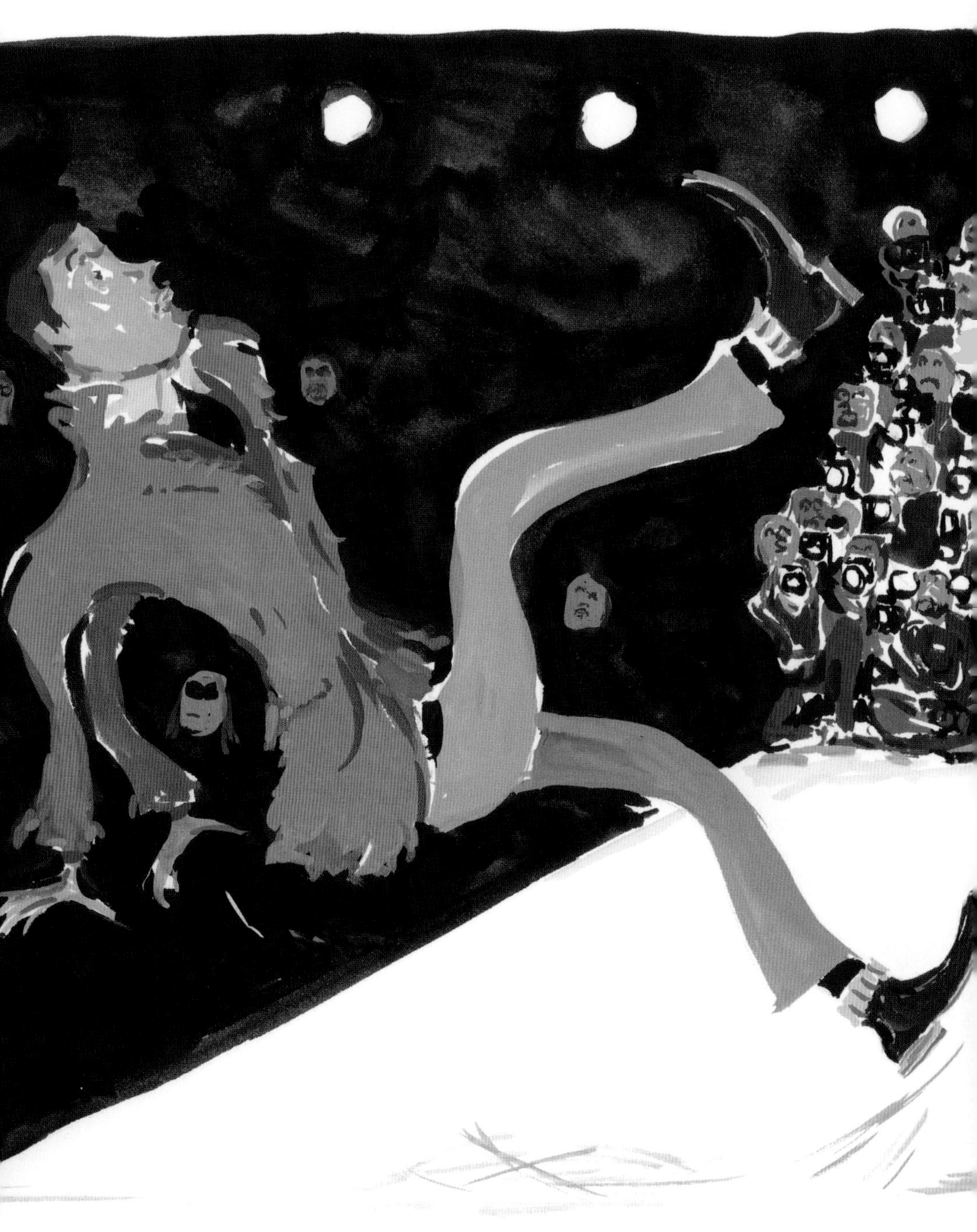

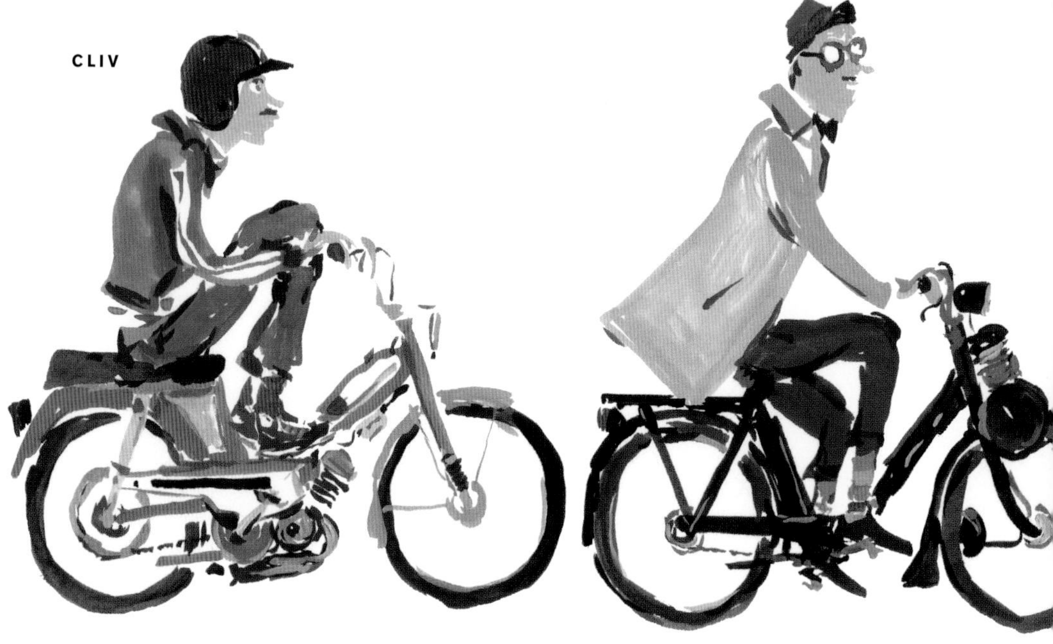

VII —— 021

HOW CAN YOU LOOK LIKE A BIKER WITHOUT THE RIDE?

The solution is simple: get your hands on a pair of motocross or mountain bike gloves. Something between Ryan Gosling's and Daft Punk's. No one's forcing you to wear them. But paired with your leather, reefer, hunting, or denim jacket, it'll be explosive.

VII —— 022

SHOULD YOU SPEAK A FOREIGN LANGUAGE WITH THE BEST POSSIBLE ACCENT?

We'd like to say yes. We'd also like to believe that people with an impeccable accent aren't annoying as hell. We'd love to help you improve your intonation, too, so you could at least express yourself properly. We'd like so many other things, but alas, it's all in vain. Do us a favor and limit yourself to a falsely unpracticed imitation of the language you are trying to speak. For your foreign friend, this inept resistance will add to your charm.

VII —— 023

What should you wear when the weather sizzles?

Forget polka-dot shirts (though they're great if you like rock) and go instead for a safari jacket with pockets, pleats, and epaulettes. Depending on the kind of guy you are, you'll look like a boy scout, Indiana Jones, or Ian Curtis from Joy Division.

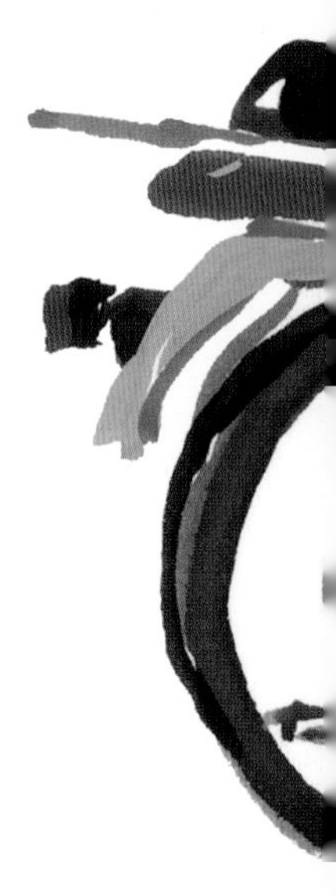

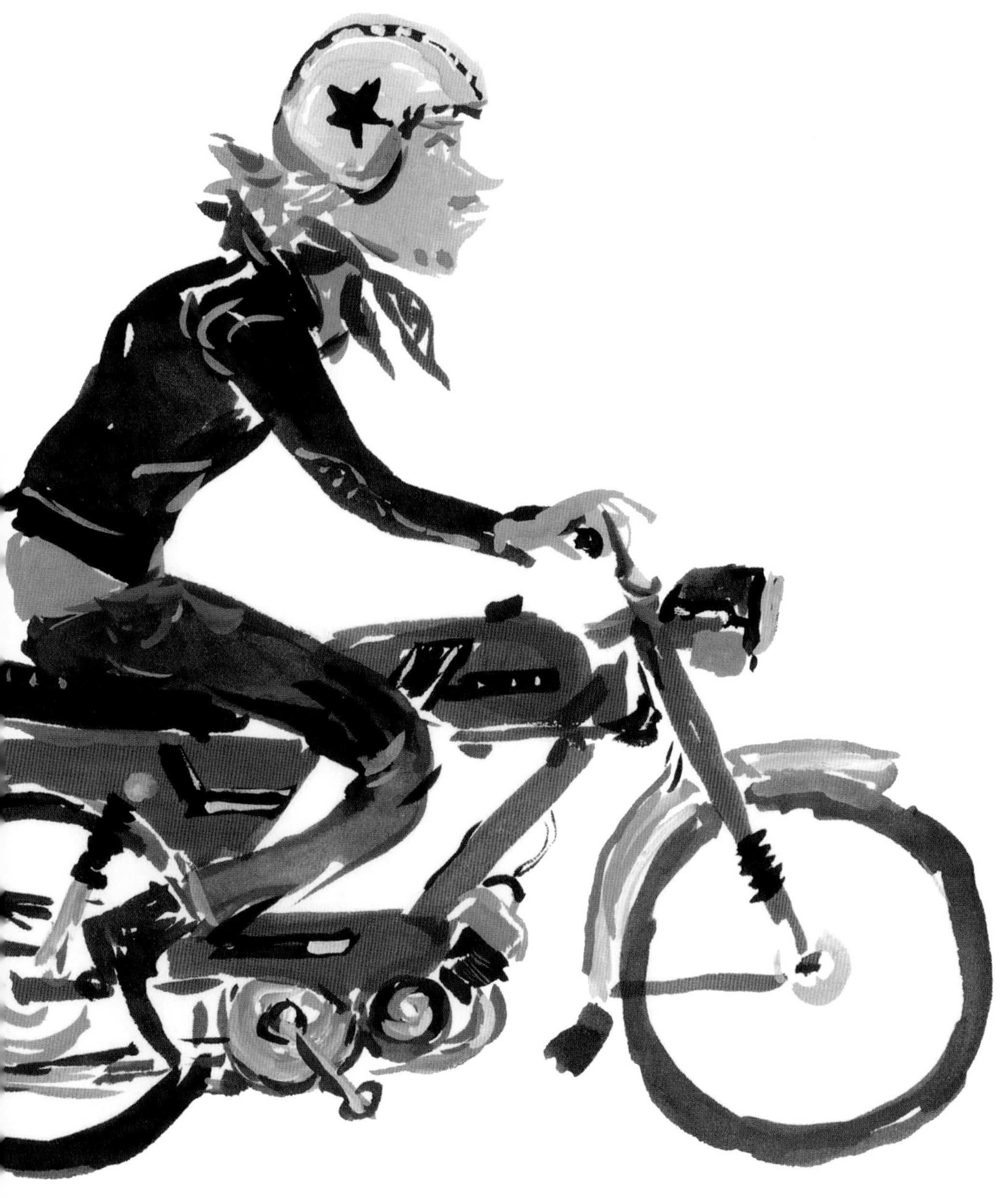

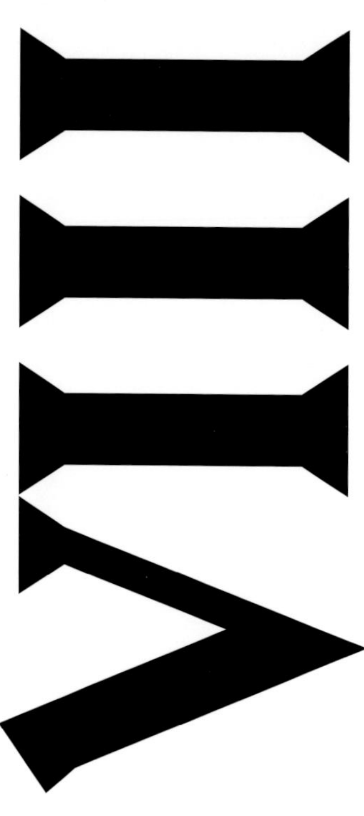

AVOID

VIII —— 001 › VIII —— 022

Can a man wear knee-high dress socks? • How should you sign off a business email? • Can you drink out of a shoe? • Should you smoke after making love? • Should you ever try fox hunting? • Are children welcome at the office? • How can you look sharp without falling flat? • How can you strike back against clingy swimwear? • Is it ok to wear fur-lined shoes? • Does your age dictate your footwear? • What should you do with your arms in beach photos? • How should you protect your

THE WORST

head from the sun's evil UV rays? • How can you keep your feet from swelling when flying? • Can you give the finger in a photo? • What's up with thick-soled shoes? • Should you join the conga line? • What is summer's greatest threat? • How do you leave a party? • What are the rules for pre-aged jeans? • Should you succumb to the tourist hotel breakfast buffet? • Should you take photos with a tablet? • Should we pay tribute to recently deceased stars?

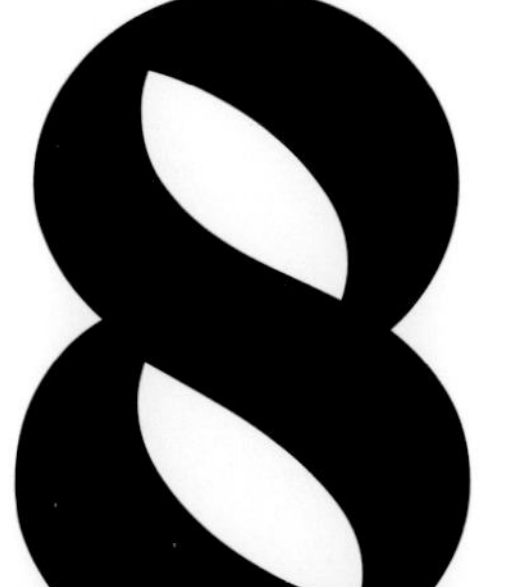

CHAPTER EIGHT

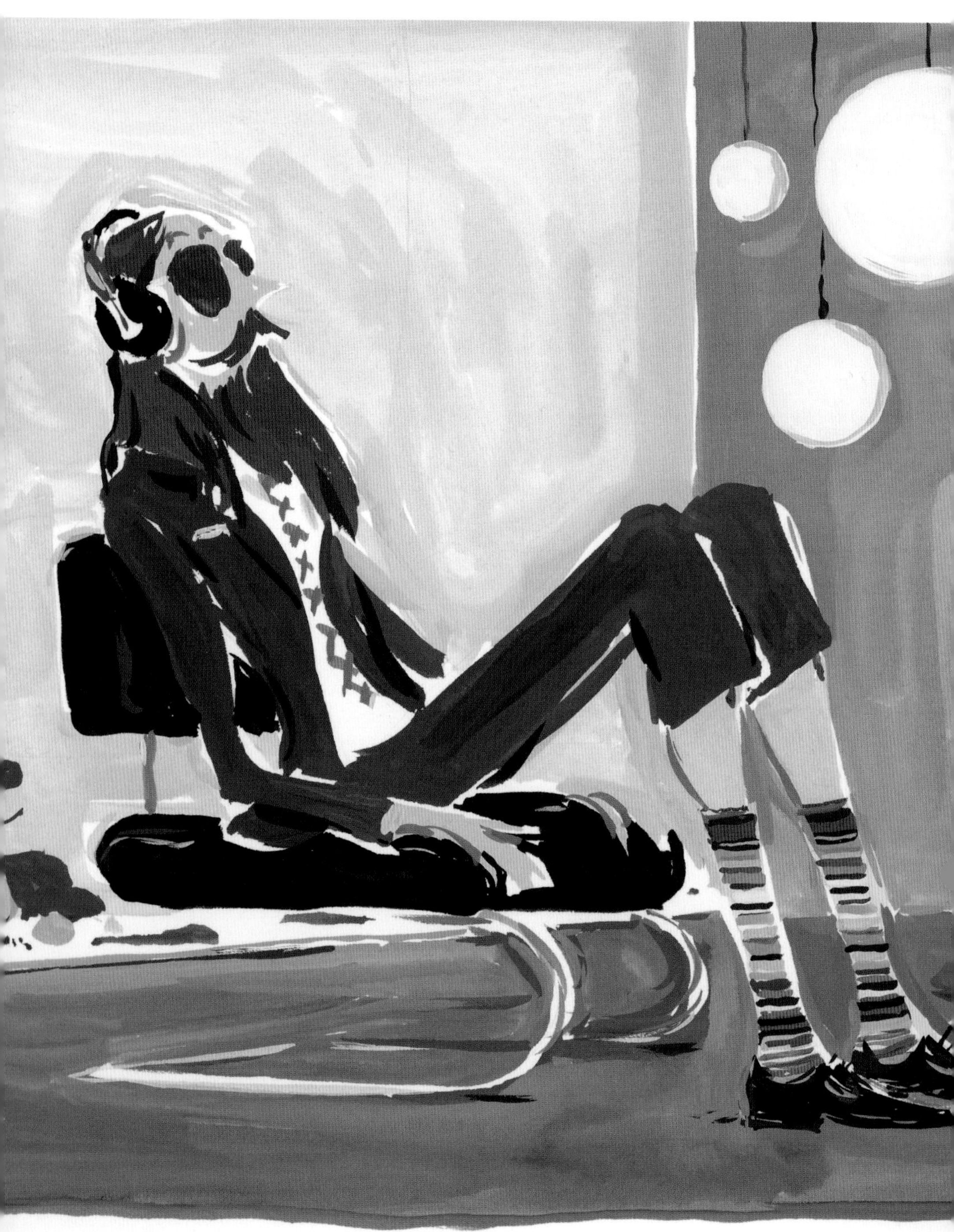

AVOID THE WORST

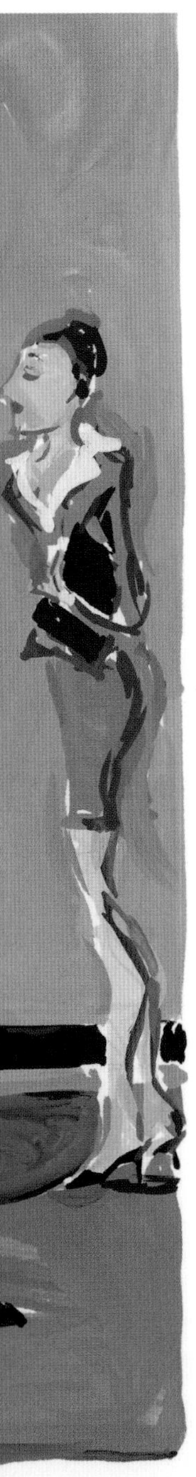

VIII — 001

CAN A MAN WEAR KNEE-HIGH DRESS SOCKS?

Like so many other questions we've addressed, this one may seem silly, but it isn't. So kindly stop thinking it is. How many times have we been deeply outraged—and we choose our words carefully here—by the sight of a seated man revealing a bit of calf? If you're wearing a suit, we encourage you to wear black or navy blue knee-high dress socks. Their innate slipperiness, just like ladies' stockings, will keep you from grousing (as you undoubtedly do) when your wool sock catches on your pant leg as you sit. When in jeans or lightweight trousers, you can forget about this issue once and for all. Pull on your knee socks, just high enough so that no one will catch a glimpse of your bulging calves. It goes without saying that any pair whose elastic has given up should go straight into the garbage.

VIII — 002

HOW SHOULD YOU SIGN OFF A BUSINESS EMAIL?

When calling cards—on which you could easily write up to two of your most elegant sentences—were de rigueur, you crossed out your name printed on the card if you were on intimate terms with your correspondent. Three hundred years later, not much has changed. The only difference is that, in some professions, your electronic signature (like your employment contract) attests to your existence within the business. In the event of any dispute, this could come in handy. Your job title offers legal proof of your position in the organizational chart of this fine company that chose you, because you were you and it was it. And that's that.

VIII —— 003

CAN YOU DRINK OUT OF A SHOE?

Yes, you can, because a shoe is just another container. For centuries, clever young rogues entertained themselves by sipping champagne from women's slippers. In more recent times, the excellent Interior Lux, the lead singer of The Cramps, took a stab at doing it onstage. The method is simple, but it must be followed closely. Take hold of your friend's high heel (remove the foot first), with the toe of the shoe tilted upward. Pour the equivalent of two or three sips of the beverage in question into the heelpiece (a note to novices: the heel doesn't taste the same as the toe). The liquid thus maintains most of its gustatory features. Take your time trying it before moving on to another diversion.

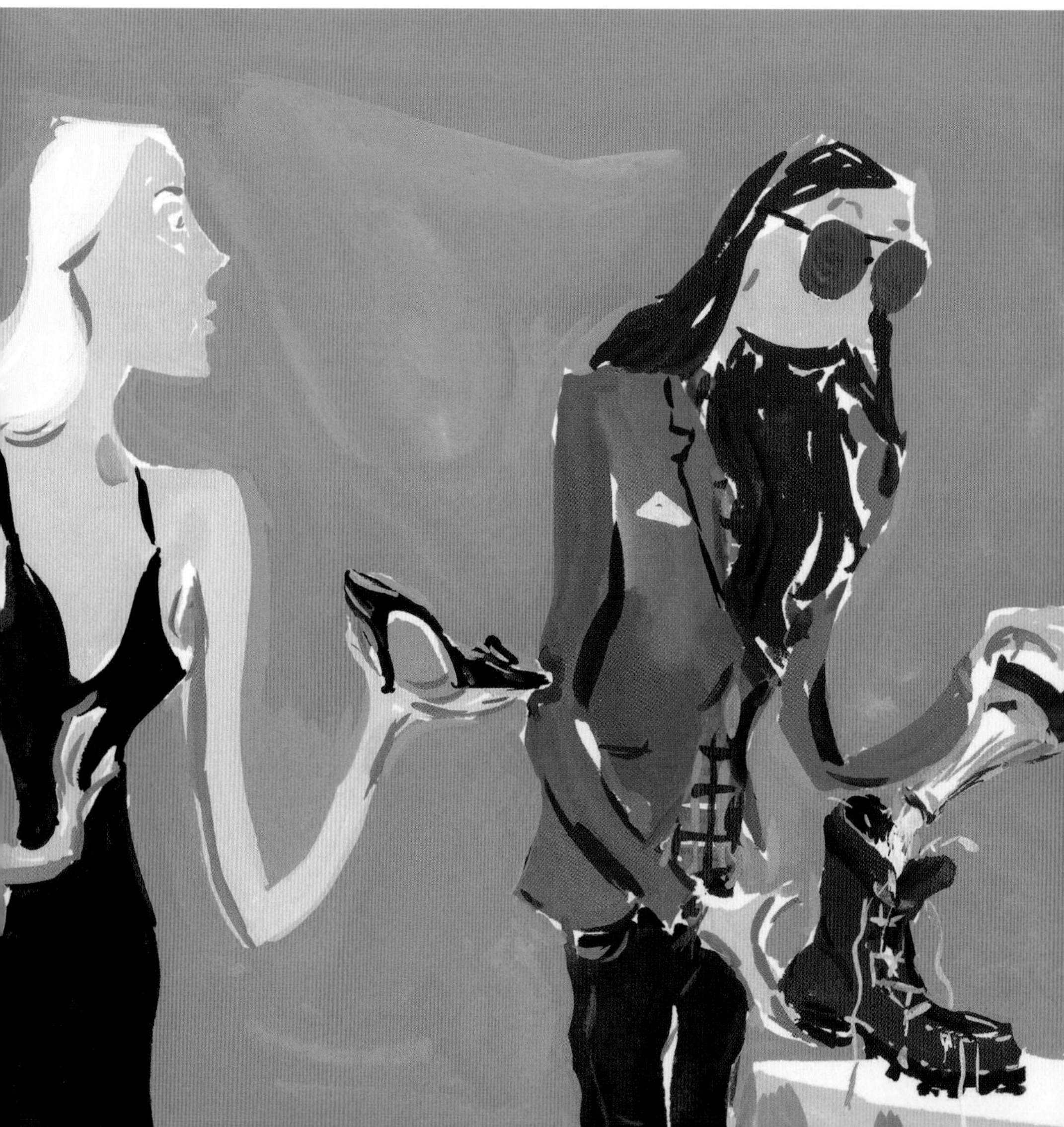

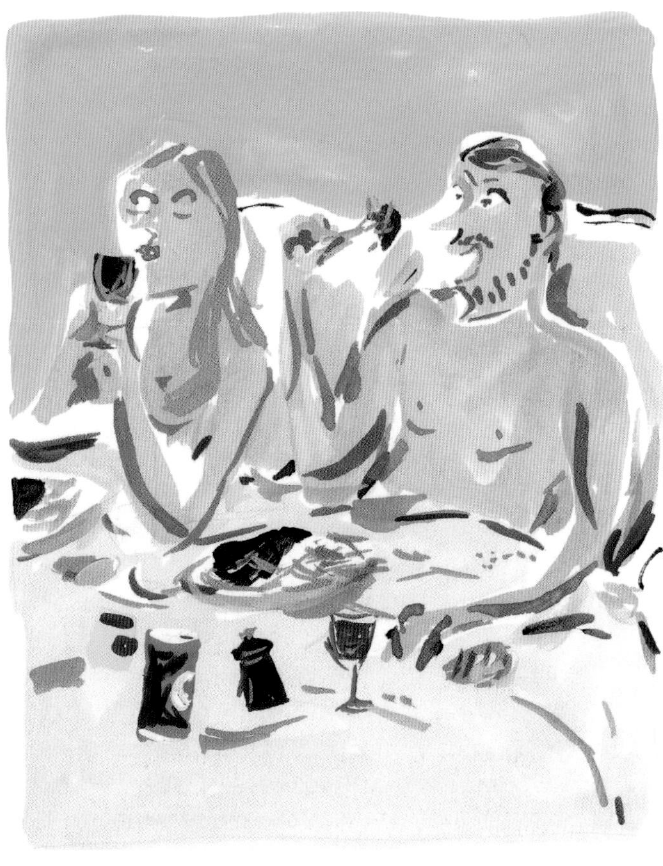

VIII —— 004

SHOULD YOU SMOKE AFTER MAKING LOVE?

If you're used to congratulating the mistress of the house with a hearty and resounding belch after an excellent dinner, then don't hesitate to blow smoke rings over your sleeping conquest's backside. Strict rules apply here: after the act, you can't just do any old thing. Total liberty should be expressed during the act, not once the curtain falls.

VIII —— 005

SHOULD YOU EVER TRY FOX HUNTING?

If you're inclined to live dangerously, why don't you head to the zoo instead? A solid knowledge of animals is the earmark of a man of taste. And even if the signs say not to, go ahead and throw them a few nuts.

VIII —— 006

ARE CHILDREN WELCOME AT THE OFFICE?

While we all agree that children shouldn't have to enter the world of work too early, it's also true that they should not be left in a parked car when the daycare center is closed. To handle this type of situation with aplomb, teach your child how to behave as early as possible. Since other people's children are not always trouble, you have a sliver of a chance that yours will also behave tolerably. Otherwise, keep a *SpongeBob SquarePants* DVD handy and that charming babysitter on speed dial.

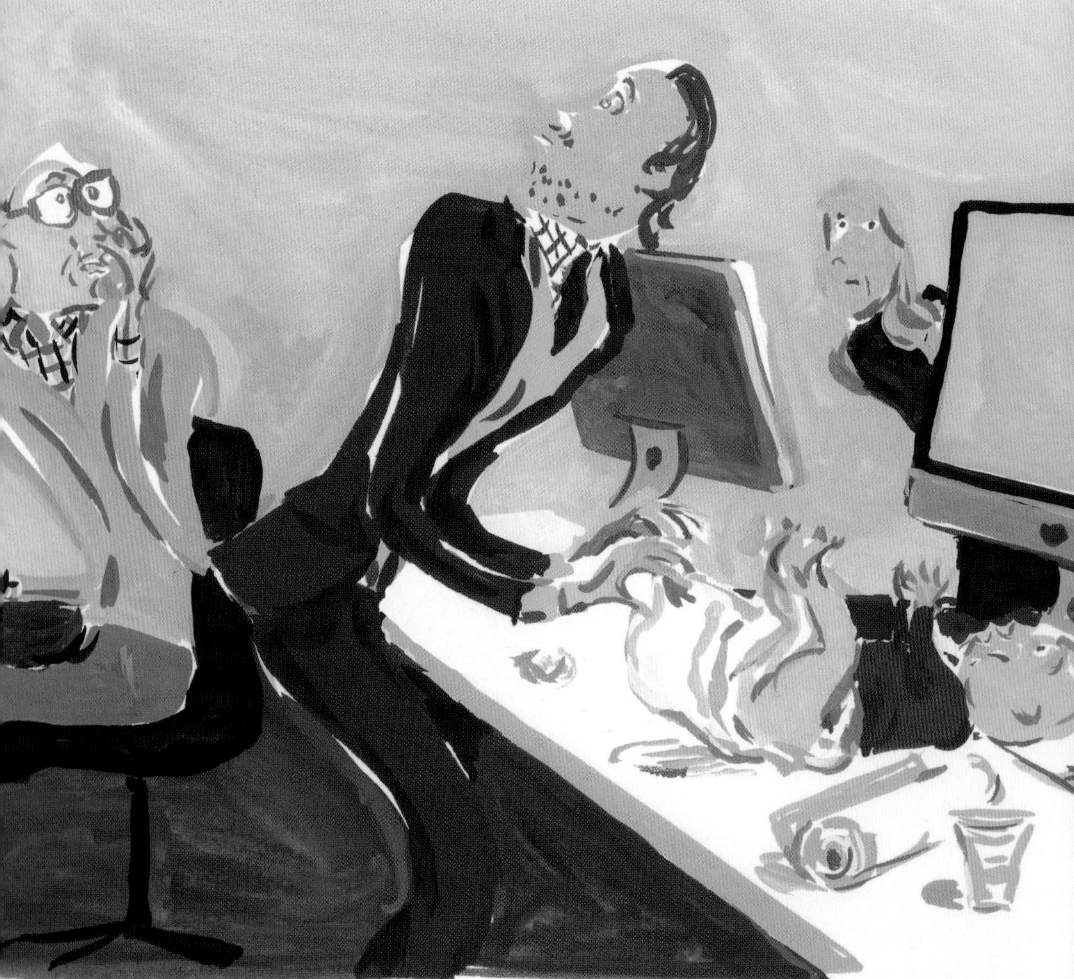

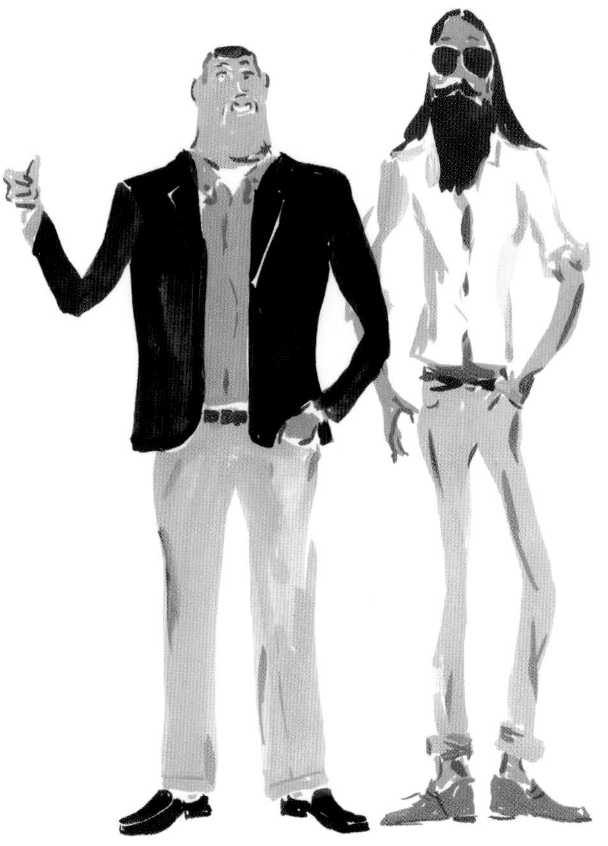

VIII — 008

How can you strike back against clingy swimwear?

Getting out of the water in a dignified manner is not easy, especially not since Daniel Craig set the bar so high in *Casino Royale*. You, the ordinary mortal, have one shot at getting it right. At this very moment, you feel like all of humanity is watching you. As expected, your swimming trunks act like a suction cup as you come out of the water. Ignore it. Let the whole beach see you as nature intended.

VIII — 007

HOW CAN YOU LOOK SHARP WITHOUT FALLING FLAT?

To avoid that square, clean-cut look, don't trim your hair too short if you are on the heavy side. The epitome of boring is to wear neat and ironed beige chinos, a button-down shirt of a blue so bland as to be considered a neutral, a roomy blazer, and a pair of black loafers to go with a new, neutral belt. If you're aiming for that all-American look, just turn the tables on the preceding parameters. Though neat, the haircut is a mix of short and long, and a three-day beard is obsessively maintained. The silhouette—somewhat younger—is less filled out. The chinos are rolled up to the ankle over a pair of desert boots. The snugger fit pants are combined with an open—but not too open—shirt, with sleeves rolled up over the elbows, whose cut follows the contours of the body. The shirttails are out, falling just past the hips.

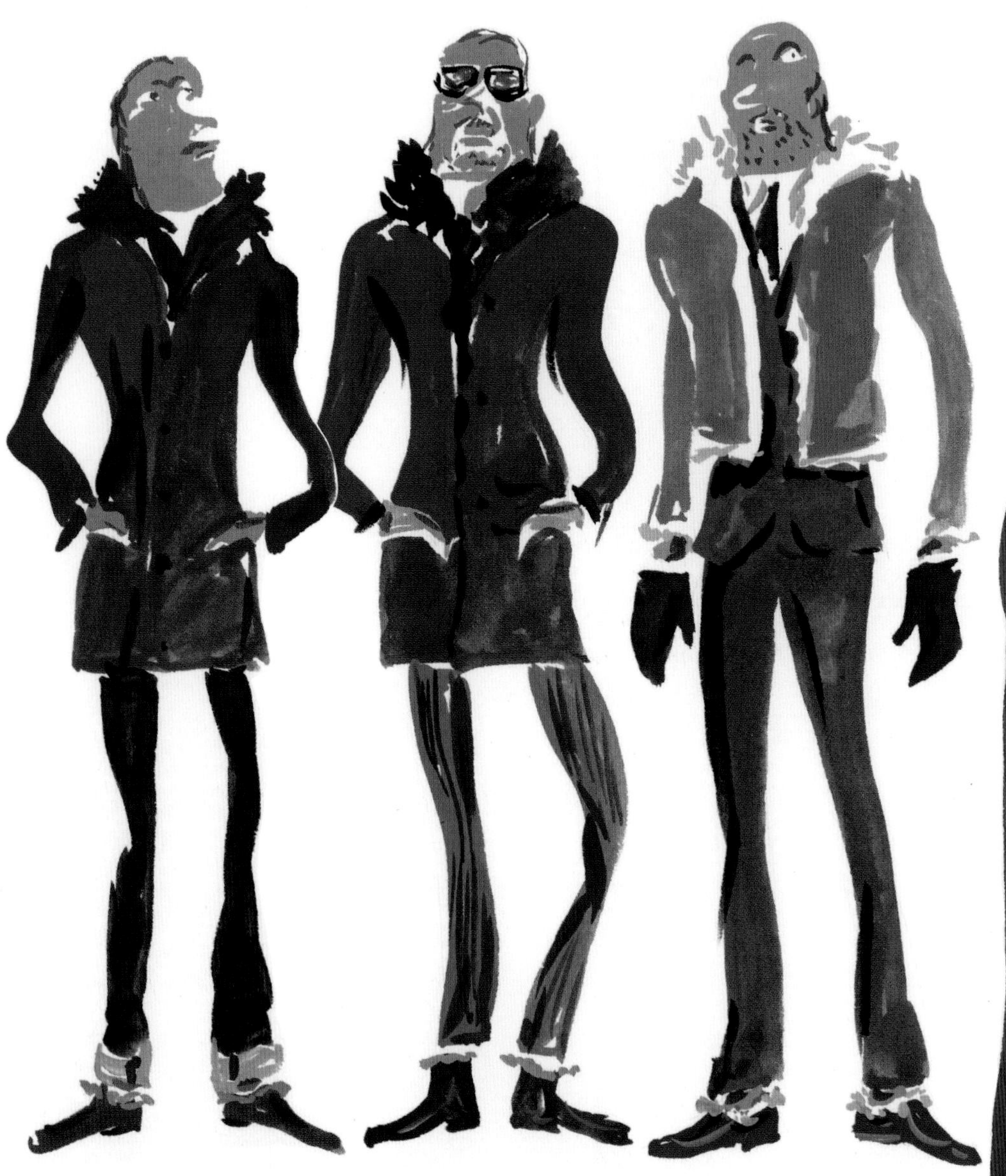

VIII —— 009

IS IT OK TO WEAR FUR-LINED SHOES?

At the back of the TV program guide, you used to see ads aimed at seniors with problem feet, in which a finger held up a lightweight bootie that even a peg leg would have refused. And now? Today, things are even worse: those awful cads even put them in the aisles of your favorite stores, prominently on display. Just between us, it's better to vaunt your love of animals somewhere else on your anatomy—around your neck, for example, since fur-collared coats and parkas are making a comeback, much to the delight of your inner dandy.

VIII — 010

DOES YOUR AGE DICTATE YOUR FOOTWEAR?

There's nothing more unusual yet appropriate than a (pre-) retired person wearing the latest sneakers. If such a person's birthday is approaching and you don't have a gift yet, give him a boost with this unexpected offering. Help him look younger for less—payback for spending your post-adolescent years trying to look older.

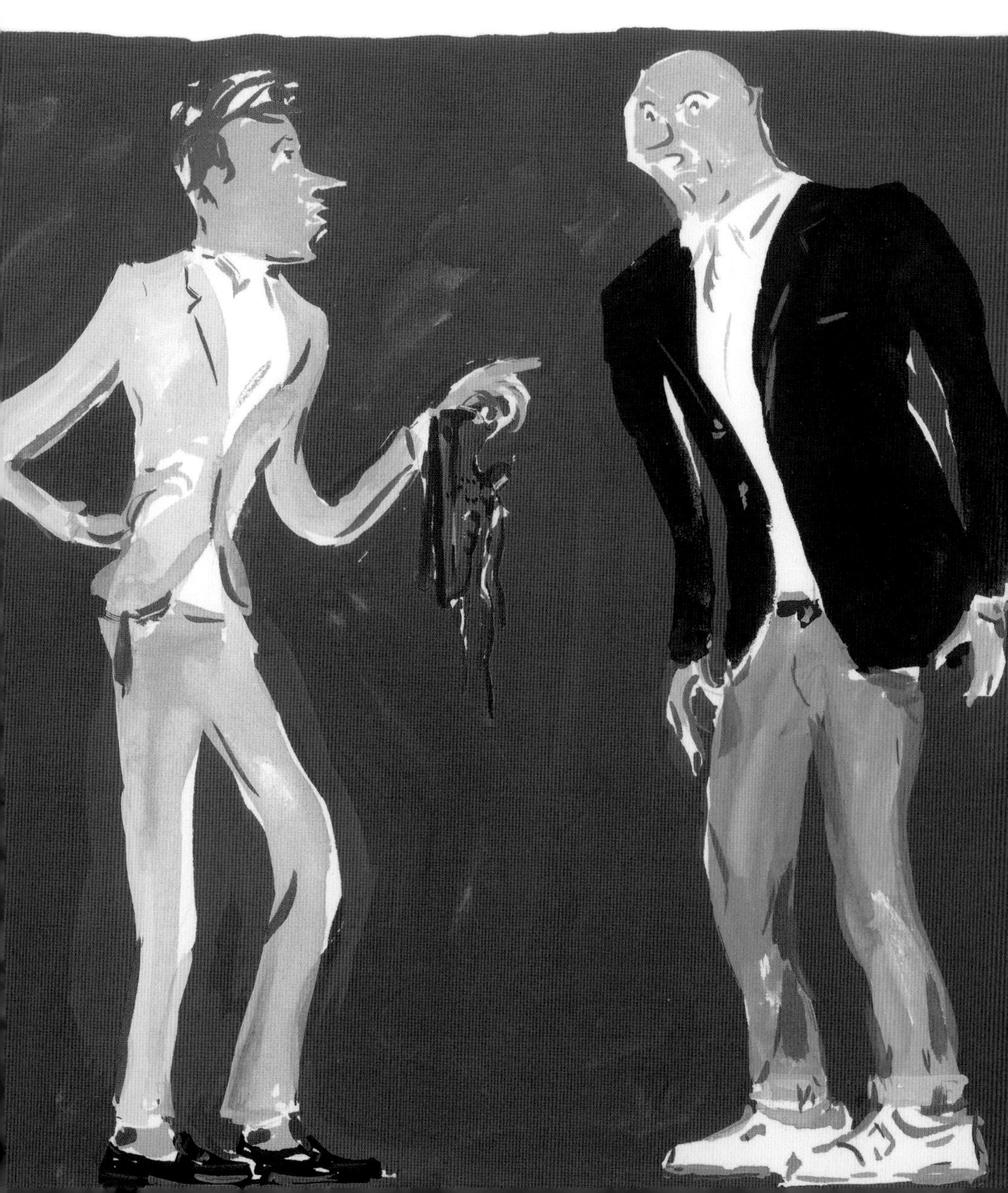

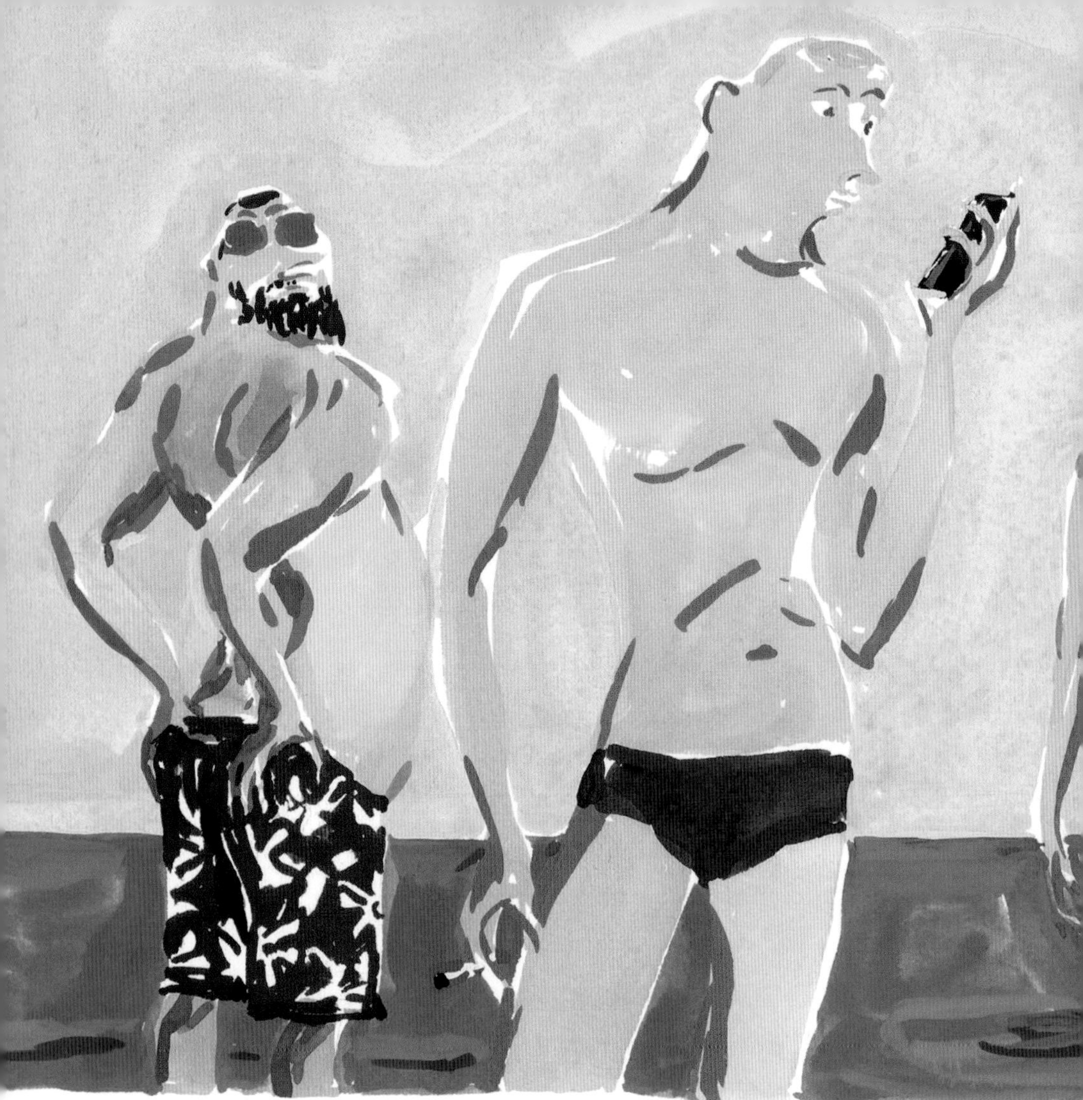

VIII —— 011

WHAT SHOULD YOU DO WITH YOUR ARMS IN BEACH PHOTOS?

Can a gentleman have his picture taken in his bathing suit, with his hands placed on his lower back? One hand works, just about, as long as it's on the hip. Both hands make you look like you're expecting. With your arms hanging by your side, you resemble a monkey (or a moron—you choose). With a towel around your neck, you look like a lifeguard. With it around your hips, people will think you're naked; any higher up and you'll look obese. Take inspiration from Michelangelo's *David*: one arm hangs, while the other, chest level, is in the middle of completing a task. In a bathing suit, a guy should be either in motion or lying down. If he is static, his arms should be doing two entirely separate things, in the most natural-looking way possible. Good luck.

VIII — 012

HOW SHOULD YOU PROTECT YOUR HEAD FROM THE SUN'S EVIL UV RAYS?

When it comes to the sun, men try to be all macho and don't wear hats. It certainly looks better in photos, of course, but these days it's pretty dumb. Unless you want to resemble an average Joe tourist—a style that is not entirely without merit—don't automatically reach for a baseball cap. You can't just wing it with a cap; it's like rock climbing or the mambo. In any event, we recommend using a beach umbrella to deal with the sun's harsh rays. After all, since you only go to the beach after five p.m., you don't need all that much protection.

VIII — 013

HOW CAN YOU KEEP YOUR FEET FROM SWELLING WHEN FLYING?

Before departure, take an aspirin to improve blood flow. Drink water throughout the trip and walk up and down the aisle a few times. Don't wear overly tight pants or they'll cut off the circulation in your thighs. Stay away from socks with elastic cuffs that will make your calves swell. Wear light, low-cut shoes: Vans or Rivieras, which will also make the security check less of a hassle. Hardcore fans of leather shoes should favor open-laced derby shoes (bucks), which have more slack than closed-laced oxfords. Otherwise, there are always support stockings. How do you think Jay-Z manages?

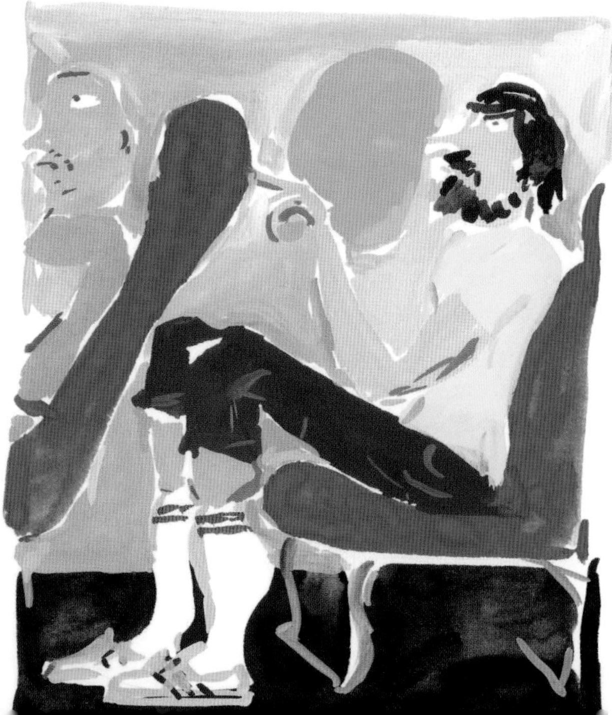

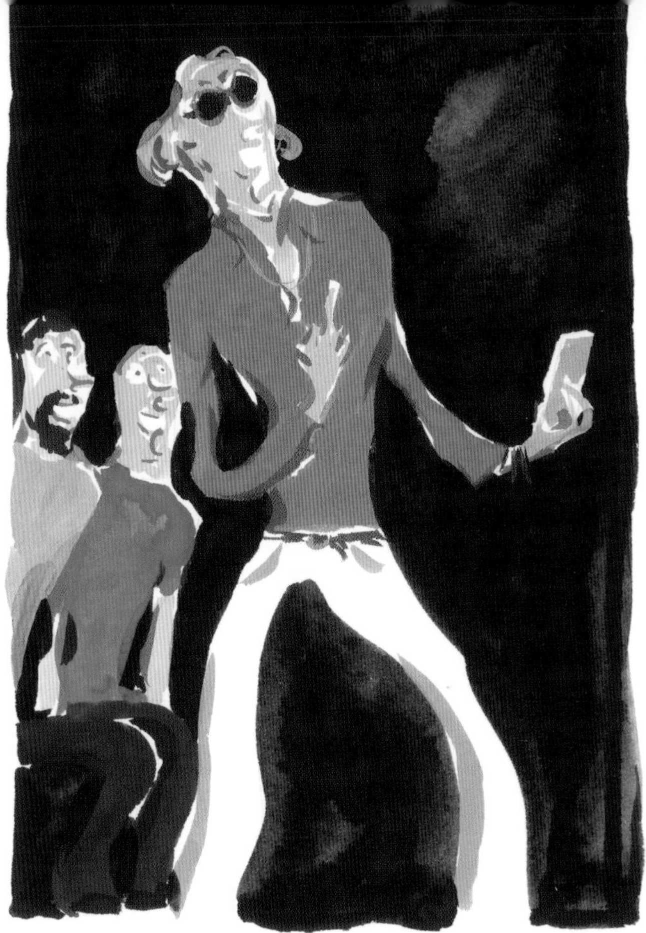

VIII —— 014

CAN YOU GIVE THE FINGER IN A PHOTO?

Flipping the bird comes in and out of fashion. Spurred on by Instagram, pop culture, and street style photographs, this year it's totally in to give somebody the finger, and it is taking over from the sidewise V used by the cool kids of yesteryear (phew!). Go for it this summer, give the finger in photos with your friends. It's important, though, to remember to do one, and only one, photo of you "flipping off." In no case should there be two. The more spontaneous the photo, the better the result.

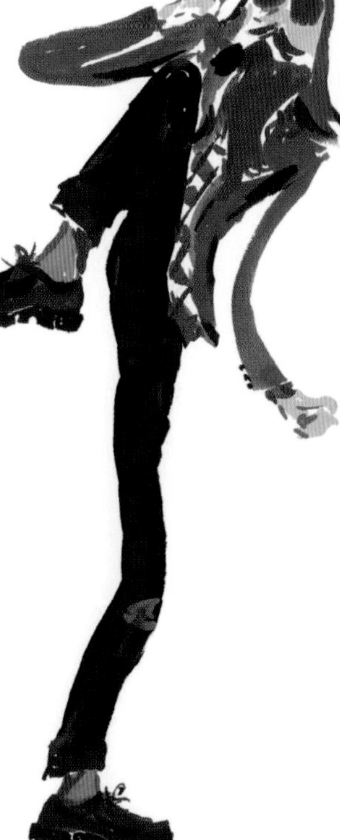

VIII —— 015

WHAT'S UP WITH THICK-SOLED SHOES?

Although they can be imposing, you might as well try the good old low-cut Paraboot model that has been ignored for such a long time (but actually seems to be coming back in style). With rolled-up corduroys, you'll be the king of winter. If someone calls you an old man, give him a kick in the privates.

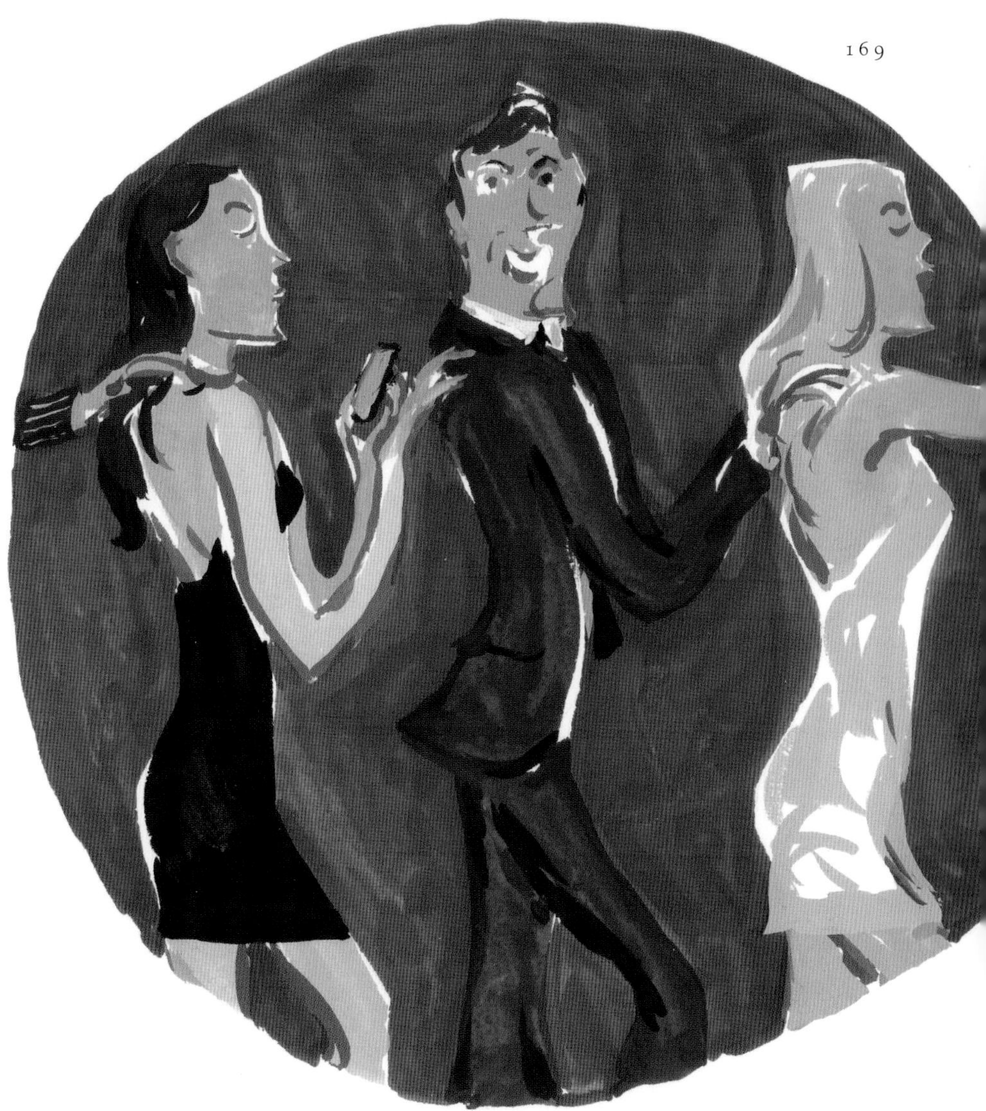

VIII —— 016

SHOULD YOU JOIN THE CONGA LINE?

Super, it's party time! The music makes the women even prettier, and the guys drinking in the corner have noticed this sudden transformation. We'd be in heaven, if only the atmosphere wasn't so stiff and everyone would just loosen up. A current hit starts playing—it's the perfect time to get an awesome conga line under way. The posers, caught in the clutches of that despot "cool," are giving you serious hairy eyeball. But once past a certain age, people start remembering what it really means to have fun.

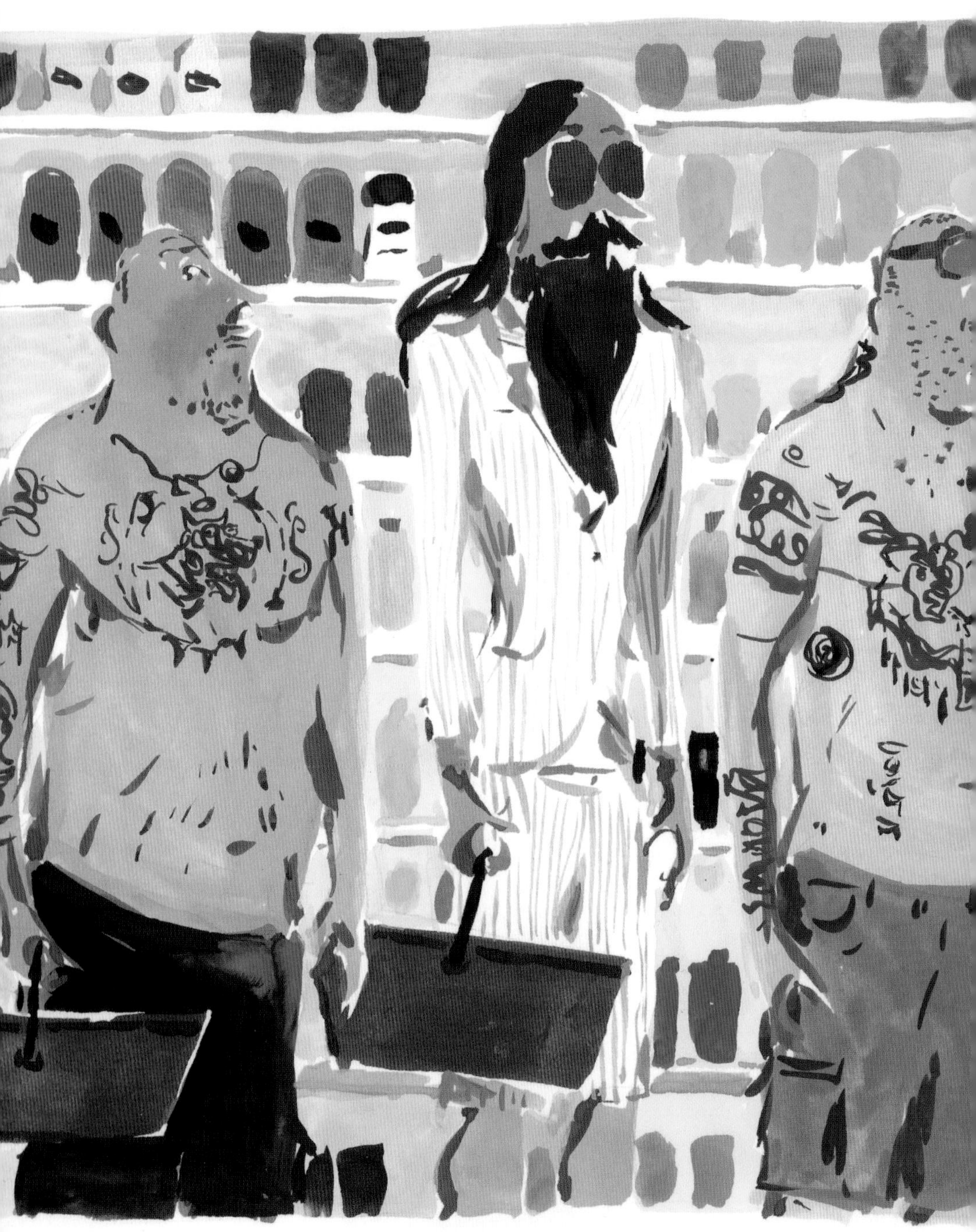

AVOID THE WORST

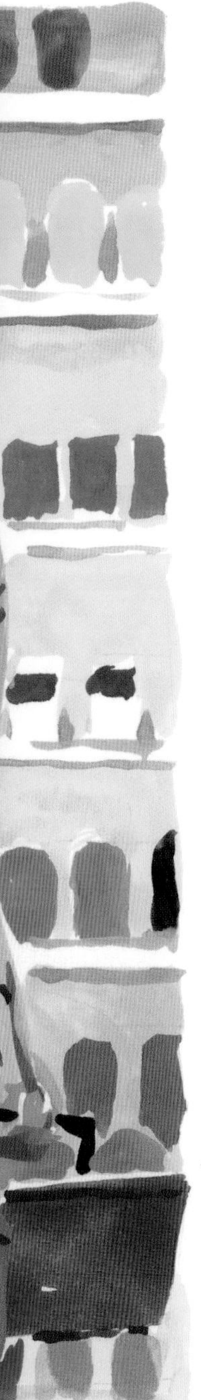

VIII — 017

WHAT IS SUMMER'S GREATEST THREAT?

Looking like an idiot in your quest for cool, that's what. Warm weather, being on vacation, and a carefree spirit spur some to go shirtless to the supermarket. While we know you wouldn't go that far, we suggest you keep unrestrained exhibitionism—a sport ordinarily reserved for children under the age of three—under wraps. What goes for your chest also goes for your feet, for two good reasons. First, flip-flops and other footwear that reveal your toes only look good on Roman legionaries and Brazilian beachgoers. Second, if you wish to show off your feet, they have to be as flawless as your teeth—and you clean those three times a day.

VIII — 018

How do you leave a party?

If you have planned your exit ahead of time, be unobtrusive from the start. Be polite and no more. If the idea comes to you all of a sudden, lay the groundwork. Become the center of attention ("You got to burn to shine," says the Beat poet John Giornio). At the high point of the party, let things cool down a bit then go to your hosts and briefly present your excuses. Disappear. Do it again somewhere else. And then somewhere else again.

VIII — 019

WHAT ARE THE RULES FOR PRE-AGED JEANS?

Yellowed jeans recall the hard-scrabble America of *Little House on the Prairie* and the novels of Cormac McCarthy (*The Road, No Country for Old Men, The Border Trilogy*). Bleached jeans, on the other hand, are more often found in the washing machine than when scraping a living from the land in Walnut Grove, and they evoke a sense of automated, urban alienation. No, seriously. Many designers today offer falsely yellowed jeans, as though yanked from the wardrobe of time, stolen from gold diggers who dug up nothing but trouble. The Japanese are particularly talented at this. That aside, and speaking as a Che Guevara of style, it's those (bleached) white lines that bring us our greatest sense of euphoria.

VIII —— 020

SHOULD YOU SUCCUMB TO THE TOURIST HOTEL BREAKFAST BUFFET?

We must admit that during the past few vacations, when even the downtimes were good, the breakfast rooms filled with hot plates of scrambled eggs, bacon, and baked beans were enough to ruin the day. The English-style cooking wasn't the problem; it was the idea (though generous) of an all-you-can-eat breakfast, a profusion that marred the exceptional character of our trip. Next time we'll choose room service. Too bad for the beans.

VIII —— 021

Should you take photos with a tablet?

Wanting to do things like the Japanese is perfectly understandable. The French, who aren't always up with the latest trends when it comes to good tourist practices, can take inspiration from them. But they should hurry, since there are something like twenty generations of tablet already out there. For years now, the world has been invaded by a plethora of amazing devices for taking photographs. To give in to the phenomenon of using a tablet today (selfie stick or not) would be the equivalent—as if a parallel were necessary to help you get the picture—of breaking into a Gangnam Style dance in three years from now.

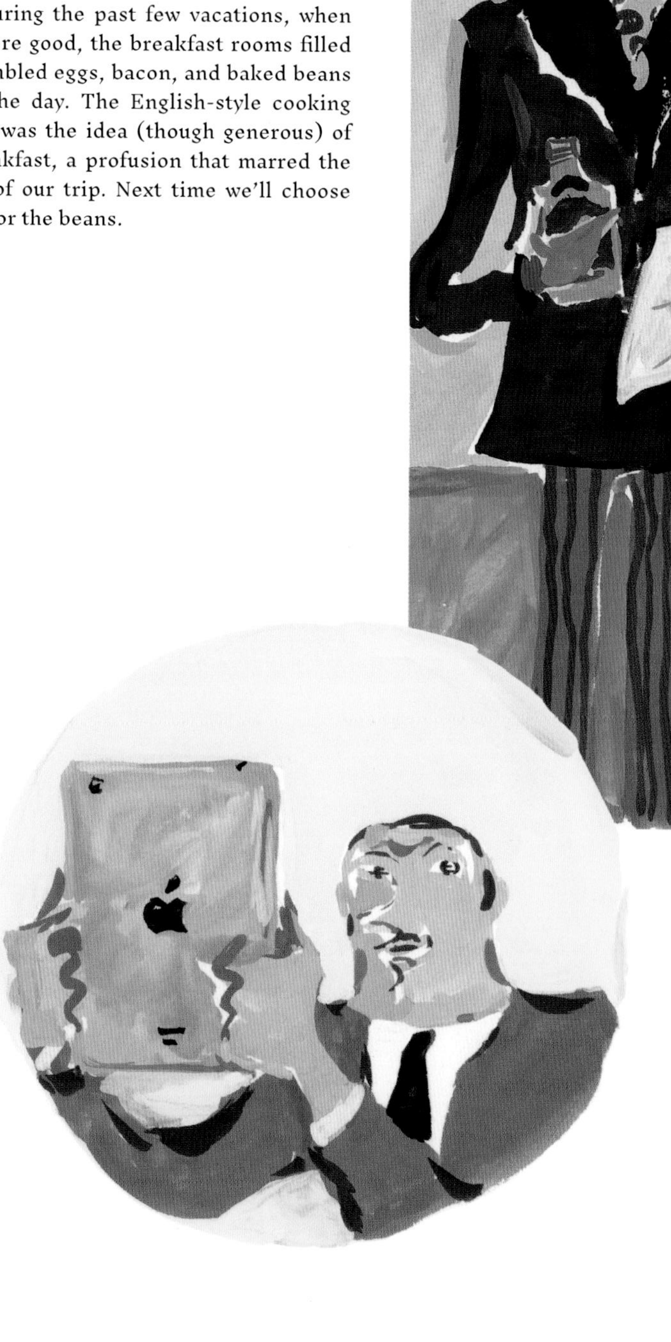

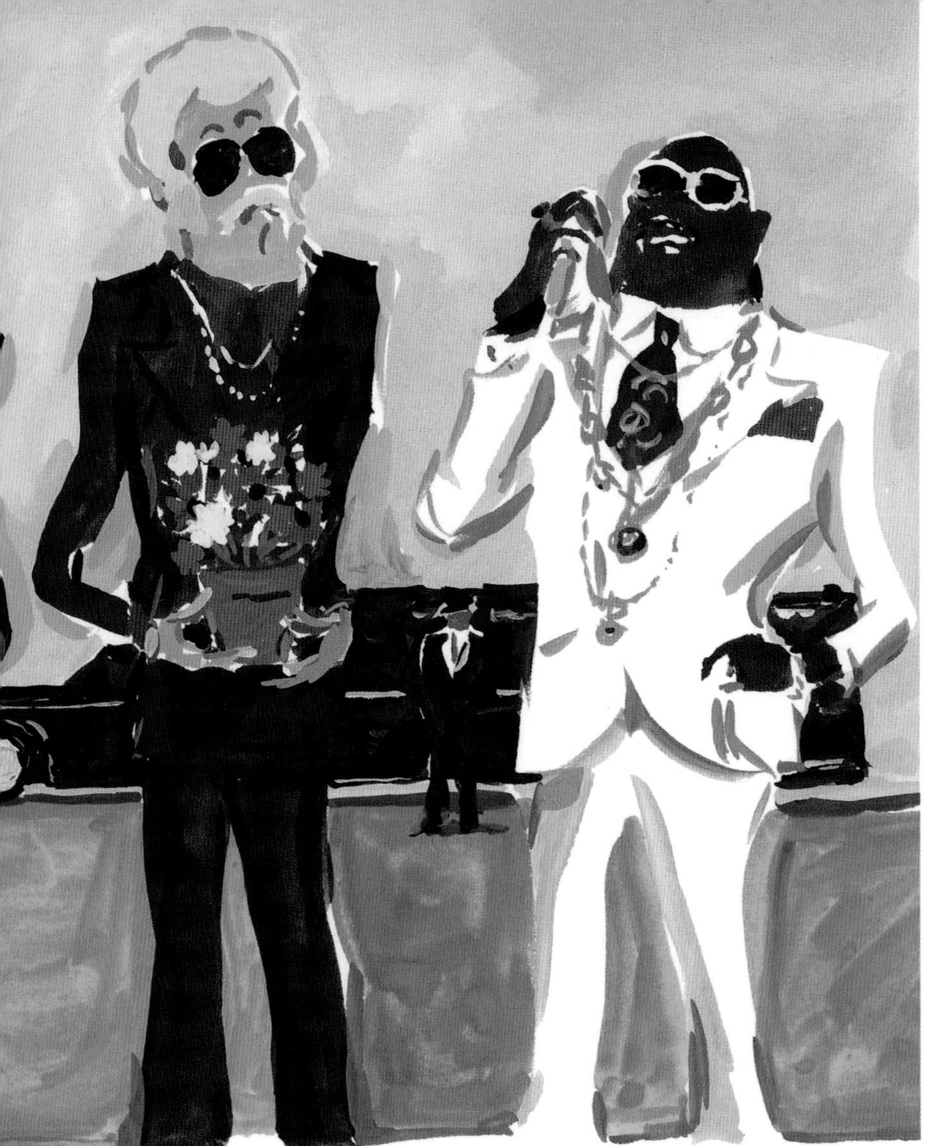

VIII —— 022

SHOULD WE PAY TRIBUTE TO RECENTLY DECEASED STARS?

They say not to speak ill of the dead. And everyone takes that to heart, literally, at the news of the death of a celebrity. The lachrymose are quick to see the hidden genius in any old has-been caught in the spotlight. The next time a poor movie or TV star dies, remember you have no reason to be personally affected by it. In any case, those whose work was praised to the skies or dragged through the mud (and sometimes both) are condemned to eternal life.

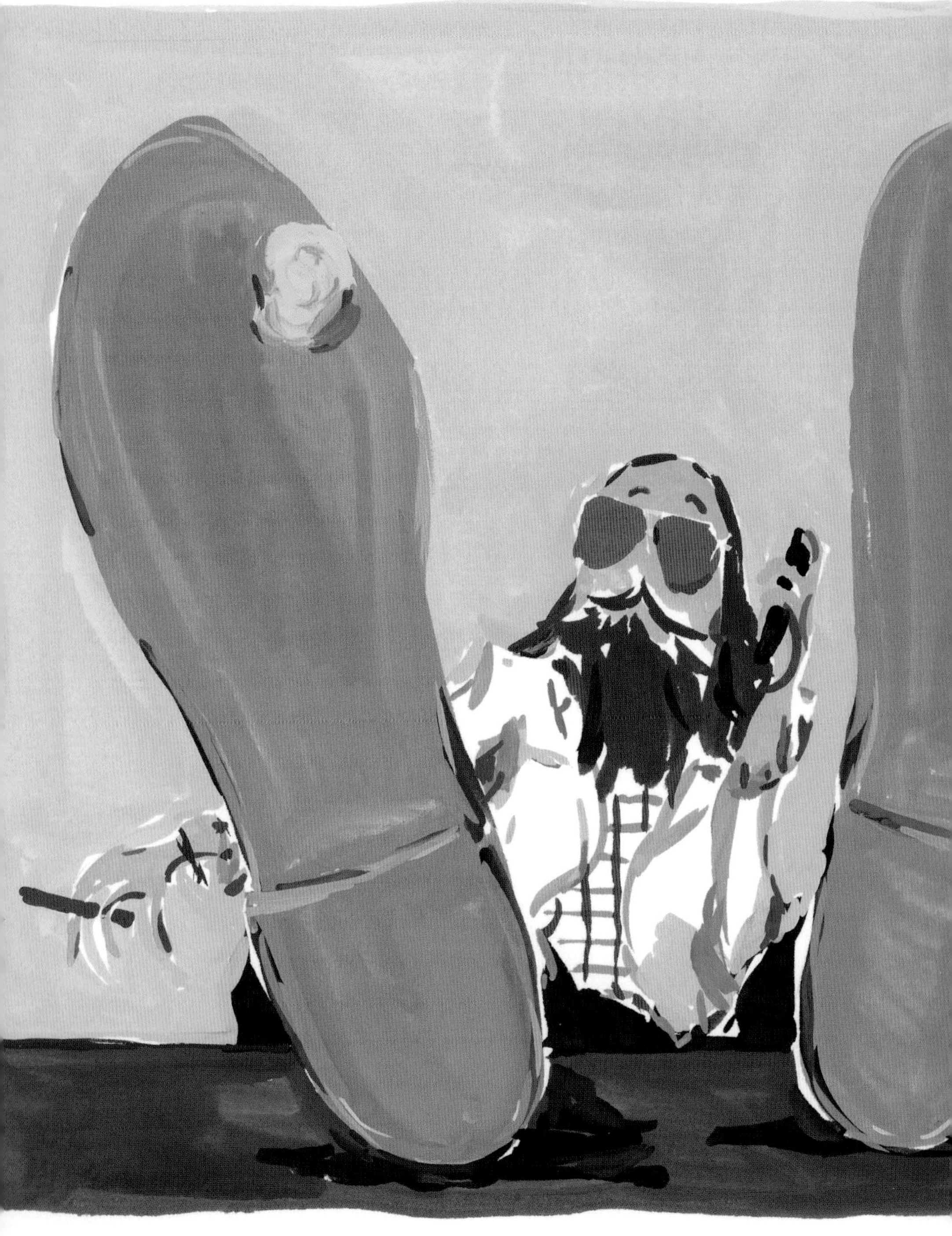

ACKNOWLEDGMENTS

Gonzague Dupleix, Jean-Philippe Delhomme, and Celya Bendjenad would like to thank Jonathan Newhouse, Xavier Romatet, Emmanuel Poncet, Louis Orlianges, and all those who have been the backbone of *GQ* since its founding, as well as Guillaume Robert.

Gonzague would also like to take this opportunity to thank his girlfriend, family, and friends.

Jean-Philippe extends his thanks to Paul Chemetoff, Anne Boulay, and his sons Joseph and Lewis—with whom he can chew over the question of hairy chests—and his friend Glenn O'Brien, the Socrates of style and what lies beyond.

Celya wishes to thank her sisters and parents, Mathieu Le Maux, the C.A.M., the Gang, Dan Lebaz, and Adrien Kissel.

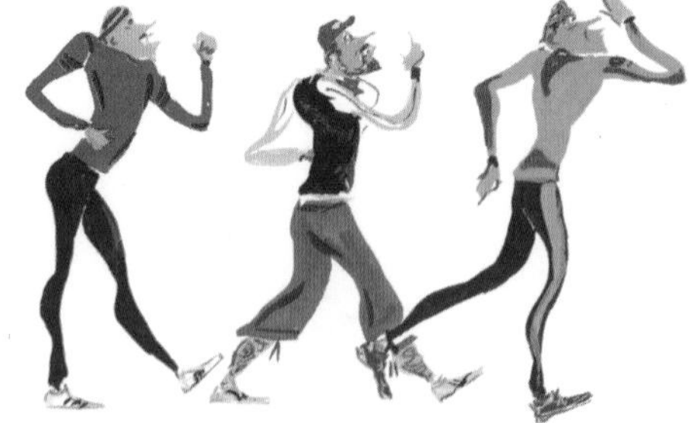